T0267362

Praise for *Waiting in Hope*

In this honest, hope-filled book, readers will find biblical truth from women who have walked a similar road. This is a beautiful reminder of God's goodness and presence for anyone walking through infertility.

Ann Swindell, author, *The Path to Peace*, owner, Writing with Grace

Infertility is isolating, heartbreaking, physically brutal, and one thousand other crushing things. Through *Waiting in Hope,* you will feel seen, encouraged, and restored. Hope will fill your heart in a season that feels pretty hopeless. While this is a topic few people talk about, Kelley and Jenn share raw and vulnerable stories. You will find yourself nodding your head as if they are sitting across from you, wiping tears away because finally someone else gets it, and laughing because they know all the ridiculous things that can be part of trying to conceive. You will feel hope again no matter what comes next in your journey. If you know someone who has experienced waiting or loss and you've never really known what to say or do, send them this book. It is exactly what they need right now!

Becky Kiser, author, speaker, life coach, founder of Online Women's Ministries

I can't think of a better descriptor for *Waiting in Hope* than "kind." As Kelley and Jenn vulnerably share their personal experiences with infertility, they lovingly validate the realities of suffering all while gently pointing the reader to Jesus. I strongly recommend *Waiting in Hope* for anyone walking the journey of infertility or for anyone who loves someone walking this road. *Waiting in Hope* is balm to a hurting heart and a guide for a weary reader toward a safe place to land.

Bobi Ann Allen, women's minister, Willowbrook Church, Huntsville, Alabama

Kelley and Jenn accurately and intimately describe the pain and loss that is infertility. *Waiting in Hope* feels like sitting on a couch with your best girl friends as they tenderly empathize with your pain and point you right back into the loving embrace of the Father. This book is a beautiful and life-giving companion for those waiting in hope for their baby.

Cathie Quillet, licensed marriage and family therapist, owner of Tennessee Reproductive Therapy, author of *Not Pregnant: A Companion for the Emotional Journey of Infertility*, The Peace (In)Fertility Workbook, *Thriving through Infertility*, and *No Matter What Happens*

As I read *Waiting in Hope*, I felt seen and known. This book is an honest conversation about the longing, grief, and suffering that mark an infertility journey. This book will give you space to grieve, tools to navigate infertility, and ultimately, help you to wait upon the Lord with hope. *Waiting in Hope* is going to be a balm for the souls of many women.

Chelsea Sobolik, author, *Longing for Motherhood*

Where can you find hope during the emotional roller coaster of waiting to build your family? Truly, it is only in discovering that "the Lord of the universe wants a relationship with you," and that ". . . the Lord's compassionate love for you will soothe your mourning heart." Kelley and Jenn, like all those experiencing infertility/recurrent pregnancy loss, didn't get to choose whether or not to travel that family building path—but they have found the secret of choosing how to travel that path by ". . . finding purpose in the One who saved (them) and sustains (their) life." Thankfully, they also chose to share their experiences and encouragement through this book of love, a resource that every infertility patient (and their partner) should read. Every corner of the journey is covered, with encouraging words from the Bible to read, reflect, pray, and act upon. Read and follow their gentle guidance through *Waiting in Hope*.

Dorothy Roach, M.D., Medical Director, HART Fertility Clinic, Houston, Texas

Kelley Ramsey and Jenn Hesse have walked the hard path of infertility—so they offer tested wisdom. They have borne the pain of uncertainty, disappointment, and loss—so they offer knowing compassion. But, most importantly, they have walked this road with Jesus—so they offer genuine hope. *Waiting in Hope* is wise, compassionate hope for the infertility journey.

Eric Schumacher, author of *Ours: Biblical Comfort for Men Grieving Miscarriage*

As a pastor, I've seen the devastation infertility can wreak on a person's faith, marriage, and life. I've also watched God move people from grief and hopelessness to joy and renewed purpose through the ministry of Waiting in Hope. Now, with the *Waiting in Hope* book, women have even greater access to life-changing support. Based in compassion and truth, this beautiful devotional is a must-read for any woman or couple who is facing or has dealt with infertility. I also encourage fellow pastors to recommend *Waiting in Hope* as a resource for ministering to your people who are walking through this challenging season.

Jason Shepperd, founder and pastor, Church Project, The Woodlands, Texas

Kelley and Jenn are your friends as you live in the land of the middle. You will be able to breathe deeper and hope bigger because of their vulnerability and guidance.

Krystalle Wheeler, founder and director, Lullaby of Hope

This is the book I wish I had when my own infertility and pregnancy loss story began. With refreshing honesty and sound truth, Kelley and Jenn remind us that it is a good idea to hope not because of what we receive, but because of who we receive. I am personally thankful for this resource and am eager to recommend it again and again.

Nicole Zasowski, licensed marriage and family therapist, author, *What If It's Wonderful?*

Has your heart been crushed by the weight (and wait) of infertility? *Waiting in Hope* is the book you need as your companion. Although I am not happy you are on this journey, I am happy that you are about to open this devotional. It will be a balm to your heart. You will hold tight to this book and revisit it again and again. Jenn and Kelley grasp your hands to figuratively join you on the roller coaster of emotions, spiritual wonderings, and relational needs that come with infertility and loss. Their gentle words remind you that you are not alone on this journey. You are loved. You are the daughter of the King. This is THE book for those who face infertility; it provides much-needed information to help calm your soul, relatable support so you know you are not alone, and the peaceful comfort of biblical wisdom for you to apply in your life. Start the journey of releasing the weight off your shoulders by reading this book today. *Waiting in Hope* is nothing short of life-changing for those with waiting hearts.

Sarah Philpott, author of *Loved Baby: 31 Devotions Helping You Grieve and Cherish Your Child After Pregnancy Loss*

For those navigating the difficult and lonely journey of infertility, *Waiting in Hope* is like a balm to the longing heart. In an honest and real way, Jenn and Kelley come alongside the reader with a beautiful blend of truth and hope. If you or someone you love is longing for a child, you will find the comfort of those who understand and the gift of gospel hope on the pages of this book.

Sarah Walton, coauthor of *Hope When It Hurts* and *Together Through the Storms*, author of *Tears and Tossings*

There are very few biblical resources for women and men facing the often-unexpected journey of infertility. Kelley and Jenn have woven stories of deep vulnerability, solid biblical truths, and practical application, shifting the narrative from isolation, pain, and loss to community, lament, and hope. Their authenticity, humility, and raw hope in Christ is beautifully displayed on the pages of these 31 reflections. As someone who frequently intersects with families walking through infertility while simultaneously considering adoption or foster care, I cannot recommend this resource enough.

Toni Steere, director, Legacy 68:5, Houston's First Baptist Church

WAITING
IN
HOPE

31 Reflections for Walking with God
Through Infertility

✧

KELLEY RAMSEY & JENN HESSE

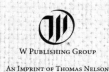

W PUBLISHING GROUP

AN IMPRINT OF THOMAS NELSON

© 2023 Kelley Ramsey and Jenn Hesse

All rights reserved. No portion of this book may be reproduced, stored in a retrieval system, or transmitted in any form or by any means—electronic, mechanical, photocopy, recording, scanning, or other—except for brief quotations in critical reviews or articles, without the prior written permission of the publisher.

Published in Nashville, Tennessee, by W Publishing, an imprint of Thomas Nelson.

Thomas Nelson titles may be purchased in bulk for educational, business, fund-raising, or sales promotional use. For information, please email SpecialMarkets@ThomasNelson.com.

Unless otherwise noted, Scripture quotations are taken from the Holy Bible, New International Version®, NIV®. Copyright © 1973, 1978, 1984, 2011 by Biblica, Inc.® Used by permission of Zondervan. All rights reserved worldwide. www.zondervan.com. The "NIV" and "New International Version" are trademarks registered in the United States Patent and Trademark Office by Biblica, Inc.®

Scripture quotations marked AMP are from the Amplified® Bible (AMP). Copyright © 2015 by The Lockman Foundation. Used by permission. www.Lockman.org.

Scripture quotations marked CSB are from the Christian Standard Bible®. Copyright © 2017 by Holman Bible Publishers. Used by permission. Christian Standard Bible® and CSB® are federally registered trademarks of Holman Bible Publishers.

Scripture quotations marked ESV are from the ESV® Bible (The Holy Bible, English Standard Version®). Copyright © 2001 by Crossway, a publishing ministry of Good News Publishers. Used by permission. All rights reserved.

Scripture quotations marked MSG are from THE MESSAGE. Copyright © 1993, 2002, 2018 by Eugene H. Peterson. Used by permission of NavPress. All rights reserved. Represented by Tyndale House Publishers, a Division of Tyndale House Ministries.

Scripture quotations marked NKJV are from the New King James Version®. Copyright © 1982 by Thomas Nelson. Used by permission. All rights reserved.

Scripture quotations marked NLT are from Holy Bible, New Living Translation. © 1996, 2004, 2015 by Tyndale House Foundation. Used by permission of Tyndale House Ministries, Carol Stream, Illinois, 60188. All rights reserved.

Scripture quotations marked TLB are from The Living Bible. Copyright © 1971. Used by permission of Tyndale House Publishers, a Division of Tyndale House Ministries, Carol Stream, Illinois 60188. All rights reserved.

Italics added to Scripture quotations are the authors' emphasis.

Some personal names and identifying details have been changed to protect the privacy of the individuals involved.

The information provided in this book does not constitute professional advice and is not a substitute for expert medical advice. When a doctor's advice to a particular individual conflicts with advice provided in this book, that individual should always follow the doctor's advice.

Any internet addresses, phone numbers, or company or product information printed in this book are offered as a resource and are not intended in any way to be or to imply an endorsement by Thomas Nelson, nor does Thomas Nelson vouch for the existence, content, or services of these sites, phone numbers, companies, or products beyond the life of this book.

ISBN 9780785290384 (Hardcover)
ISBN 9780785290414 (eBook)
ISBN 9780785290421 (Audiobook)

Library of Congress Control Number: 2022048774

Printed in the United States of America

23 24 25 26 27 LBC 5 4 3 2 1

To the woman reading this book, though you might feel hope slipping away, you aren't hopeless. You have a Friend who waits with you. We're here for you too.

To our Waiting in Hope community, you brought this resource to life. It's an honor to share your stories of walking with God through infertility.

Contents

Leaning on Hope: The Relational Journey

Walking with Hope: Journeying Forward

INTRODUCTION

Your Source of Hope

Dear friend, waiting is painful. You know this. You've felt the ache sharpen every month that passes without a baby in your arms.

We understand and are so sorry you're facing these struggles. Trying to navigate the wait for a child can be a lonely journey. Few people understand what it's like to obsess over menstrual charts or inject fertility shots into your belly or toss box after box of negative pregnancy tests into the trash.

We're sad that you're hurting, but we're glad you chose to pick up this book. Taking this step shows that you're looking for a source of hope.

The Waiting

The strange thing about waiting is that it forces us to go somewhere with our pain. While we might feel stuck in limbo, the desperation to find relief actually propels us into motion, seeking strength greater than our own.

No matter your belief system, at some point, your journey of waiting for a child will intersect with your journey of faith. This book can be your companion on that journey. We won't give you answers to every question you have or fill you with empty promises God's Word never makes. Instead, we'll be the friends who understand your sorrow, comfort you with care, and remind you of truth.

We can understand and write about these struggles because we've lived them. Our individual journeys of waiting may be different, but they mirror the same themes. In many ways, we continue to relive our seasons of infertility using the wisdom we learned then to guide us now. And we believe you can gain the same life-giving wisdom as you travel along this hard path.

Jenn's Story

I had it all planned out in college: get married, have two biological kids, then adopt two kids. My grand scheme started off on the right track when I met and married my husband. But the plan quickly fell apart when we began trying to grow our family. Besides not getting pregnant, I would suffer from excruciating cramps that lasted all month. Doctors performed several tests and two surgeries to repair my uterus and remove endometriosis. With desperation setting in, my husband and I turned to fertility treatments, going through eight rounds of unsuccessful intrauterine inseminations and a failed in vitro fertilization (IVF) cycle.

During that time, my husband and I began pursuing domestic adoption. Two months after our IVF devastation, we submitted our profile to a birth mother who had just delivered a baby boy. The next day we picked up our son from the hospital and became parents overnight. Less than two years later, God surprised us again. I got pregnant naturally and gave birth to our second son. Fast-forward seven years. Upon hitting forty, I assumed God had run out of miracles. But he wasn't done. I got pregnant a second time and delivered our third son in 2021, the same year Kelley and I started writing this book. Our family is thankful and in awe of the Lord.

My story shows God's faithfulness despite my doubt. As I wrestled with how God wasn't fulfilling my desires when and how I wanted, he gave me grace to persevere and a passion for encouraging others, prompting me to start a local infertility and infant loss support group. Even after God brought me children, he has used seasons of waiting to draw my heart toward him.

Kelley's Story

I wasn't as surprised as most women are to discover I had fertility issues. From an early age, I'd sensed deep down that my desire to be a mother would be hard to fulfill. Having painful periods since adolescence and a mother with a history of miscarriages meant my prognosis looked bleak. After seven months of negative tests, my ob-gyn sent me to a fertility specialist. He diagnosed me with low estrogen and anovulation, propelling me onto a path of impossible-to-decipher medical jargon and procedures.

Believing that I wasn't the only one struggling with these issues, I asked my church for help. We began a women's support group with two friends who were also facing infertility. I was thankful to no longer be alone and have a community of sisters who understood me.

My life has been a fast track through pain, trials, and worst-case scenarios. Yet God was always near, whispering *I'm here. Do you trust me?* By God's grace I've lived through twenty-two years of chronic pain, infertility, three miscarriages, two miraculous children conceived without treatments, and a delivery with severe complications. Today, my family and I are closer to God and pursuing our dream of adopting another child.

Through starting Waiting in Hope Ministries, I've experienced healing in my heart. It has been an honor to walk alongside thousands of women and couples during the past ten years. I continually lead them toward this healing, knowing it will affect every area in their lives. My infertility story prepared me for hardships and unknowns in a way nothing else could.

Your Story

We desire to be the friends you feel like you know, even though we've never met. We would love for you to connect with us and hundreds of women through our Waiting in Hope community. Whether you're waiting alongside your spouse or as a single woman longing for marriage and motherhood, we want you to know you're not alone. During our years of infertility ministry, we've witnessed women from all walks and seasons of life embrace their wait, allowing the hard circumstances to shape them into beautiful new creations in Christ. That's our desire for you as you read this book.

The thirty-one chapters are divided into four sections leading you through the emotional, spiritual, and relational aspects of the waiting journey, followed by thoughts to consider as you continue forward and find resolution in your waiting. Each chapter includes reflection questions, a prayer prompt, and journaling space. You may choose to read the whole book in thirty-one days, but don't feel pressured to rush. Maybe read a few chapters this month, then more next month and the month after. Linger in a chapter or section if you need time to think about a specific topic. Go at a pace that works best for you. Read on your own, with a friend, or as part of a support group. See the "About Waiting in Hope Ministries" section at the end of this book for information on our nationwide network of support groups and church resources.

Our prayer is that this book will shine a light into the darkest corners of your struggle, revealing the glory of our Savior, who died to give you life. May you see his unfailing goodness and grasp his unfading hope.

> Wait for the LORD; be strong, and let your heart take courage; wait for the LORD!
>
> Psalm 27:14 ESV

LONGING
· FOR ·
HOPE

✦

The Emotional Journey

Aboard the Roller Coaster

Hope deferred makes the heart sick, but
a longing fulfilled is a tree of life.

Proverbs 13:12

You know that fluttery feeling you get in your stomach the night before a trip to somewhere you've never visited? The tingles of excitement that keep you lying awake in bed, daydreaming about the places you'll explore and memories you'll make in this thrilling, new-to-you world?

That's the way many of us begin the journey of adding a child to our family—brimming with anticipation of the amazing experiences we'll go through and moments we'll treasure once we reach that wonderland called motherhood. It's the next stage in life, the step most people expect after marriage. Even before we take a pregnancy test, we can't help but imagine what it will be like to cradle our baby against our chest, kiss our toddler's scraped knee, and tearfully wave goodbye to our kindergartner.

If you're like me (Jenn), you've dreamed of becoming a mother since you were a little girl, toting your dolls around wherever you went. When it came time to talk with your husband about having a baby, you jumped into the process fully invested, eager, and bursting with hope. Or perhaps you hadn't envisioned yourself as a mom and were surprised at how that desire skyrocketed when you began trying to conceive. Or maybe when you were younger, you were shocked to hear a doctor say you have a physical condition that prevents or decreases the possibility of pregnancy.

However you arrived at this place of waiting, there's no way you could have anticipated how much pain you'd go through in order to have a child. There's little any of us can do to prepare for the grief of an aching womb.

Stuck on the Ride

Infertility is a ride no one wants to get on or knows how to get off. Every month you try to conceive, hope rises and crashes, plunging your heart into despair. This is why so many of us who go through this struggle call it an emotional roller coaster. Cliché or not, I can't think of a better analogy to describe it. The dizzying loop-de-loops of fertility testing. The twists and turns of navigating which options you and your husband are willing to try. The stomach-churning drop that comes after you start a new treatment, wait two grueling weeks, then see the dreaded result: *not pregnant*. It's all the emotional highs and lows of a thrill ride, minus the fun.

Why do we do this to ourselves? Anyone else would jump off this crazy coaster—not choose to hop on it again and again.

The Bible helps explain why we keep throwing ourselves into the cycle of trying to conceive and have a child. In the beginning, when God formed the universe, he breathed life into human beings with a specific blueprint: "So God created mankind in his own image, *in the image of God he created them*; male and female he created them" (Genesis 1:27). God made men and women in his image to reflect his character. As women, we're unique in that God designed female bodies to carry life. He wired us to be comforters, protectors, and caregivers just as he comforts, protects, and cares for us. Our desire to have children is good, because God instilled motherhood within the fabric of our biology.

What we don't always realize is that this good desire can become so intense that it consumes our lives. Think about your own life and the decisions you've made. Has the goal of having a baby taken over your thoughts and actions? Even now, after your hopes have been dashed cycle after cycle, you might be bracing to try another round of medication or a fertility treatment. As you grasp the faint possibility that this will *finally* be the month you'll see a second pink line, the embryos will stick, or you'll be able to carry a baby to term, you willingly subject yourself to the roller coaster while begging God to answer your prayers.

Steadfast in the Cycle

When I was stuck in the loop of trying and failing to conceive, I wrestled with the fact that God gave me a desire to have children but wasn't enabling me to get pregnant. I cried out to him, "Lord, I love you, but I don't understand. Why are you allowing this pain in my life?" I was tempted to quit after suffering years of defeat. But I didn't. I couldn't. The desire to conceive and carry a baby ran so deeply in my veins that the thought of giving up seemed as brutal as cutting off a limb.

Is this where you're at right now? Wrestling between wanting to stop the vicious cycle and not wanting to let go of your longing for a child? I know how devastating infertility is. It's a pain you can't ignore or erase. If we were sitting together, chatting over coffee or tea, I'd put my hand on yours and tell you I'm sorry. This journey is *hard*. Few other problems threaten a woman's physical, emotional, mental, and spiritual well-being more than those related to childbearing.

Though disappointment might cause you to question God's goodness, his Word assures us that he will always be our refuge in times of want and waiting.

Look at what he promises to those of us who are crying out for help:

- "The LORD is close to the brokenhearted and saves those who are crushed in spirit." (Psalm 34:18)
- "The LORD upholds all who fall and lifts up all who are bowed down." (Psalm 145:14)
- "But the eyes of the LORD are on those who fear him, on those whose hope is in his unfailing love." (Psalm 33:18)
- "For who is God besides the LORD? And who is the Rock except our God?" (2 Samuel 22:32)

God is your steady companion through the relentless letdowns of infertility. Turning to him will give you a safe landing place after your dreams collapse. As the waiting process jerks your emotions up, down, and sideways, know that the Lord your God is right there with you in the struggle. His eyes are on you, his precious daughter. His arms surround you with never-wavering love. When you're searching for strength to get through the next cycle or simply the next day, look to God as your Rock.

To Hope, or Not to Hope?

I can't tell you whether or not you should get back in line for the roller coaster. What I can guarantee is that Jesus will never leave you to ride alone. His desire to be in relationship with you remains constant through the ups and downs of trying to conceive. If you have trusted Christ for salvation, he rescued you by sacrificing himself on the cross. He redeemed you from eternal hopelessness and raised you to a beautiful, Spirit-filled life. Nothing—not even the whiplashes of infertility and waiting—can shake his love for you.

Jesus is your best hope on this turbulent journey. Let him hold you and bring comfort to your crushed heart.

Reflect

- Where are you on the roller coaster of waiting for a child? Are you feeling discouraged, stuck, exhausted, or hopeful? Take some time to name your emotions and consider how they fluctuate throughout each cycle.

_____

_____

_____

_____

_____

- Have you placed your faith in Jesus as your Lord and Savior? If not, I'd love for you to get to know him. A good starting place is to pick up a Bible and read the Gospel of John, which shares the story of Jesus' life and why he came to earth. See "How to Put Your Faith in Jesus" at the end of this book to develop a relationship that will change not only your wait but your whole life.

- If you do know and follow Jesus, are you regularly bringing your emotions before him and asking him to show you his perspective? Or are you trying to ignore, suppress, or grit your teeth through the cycles of disappointment? What, if anything, would you like to do differently in your waiting season?

_____

_____

_____

_____

_____

Pray

Dear Father, I know you're holy and good, and you created me and called me your own. Right now, my spirit feels crushed. You've given me this good desire to have a child but have yet to fulfill it. Every month, I have to endure the cycle of praying, hoping, being devastated, getting angry, feeling guilty, then asking for forgiveness. It's hard to keep trusting when I'm so tired of disappointment. Help me remember that you care and are always near. Remind me of the sacrifice Jesus paid so I could come to you and find comfort in your love. Fix my heart on who you are so I can hope even when I'm feeling let down.

Act

Go to a Bible website such as blueletterbible.org and search for characteristics of God. Then write a list of five traits that stand out to you—for example, faithful, all-powerful, gracious, compassionate, and always present. Place the list in your home, car, office, or somewhere you'll see it often as a reminder of who he is. Though the roller coaster shifts wildly, God never changes.

2

The Two-Week Wait

Peace I leave with you; my peace I give you. I do
not give to you as the world gives. Do not let your
hearts be troubled and do not be afraid.

John 14:27

What's that? A slight twinge sends my mind and heart racing. Before I (Kelley) can catch it, my imagination runs wild. *Could this be implantation cramps? My boobs hurt, don't they? Is this morning sickness I'm feeling? How soon should I take a test? Am I bloated because I'm pregnant or because I ate too much pasta last night? Why oh why do pregnancy symptoms have to be so similar to PMS?*

I wish for my sake and yours that I were exaggerating. Yet we both know how easy it is to overanalyze every little change in our bodies during the dreaded two-week wait. Nothing fills us with anxiety more than the time between when we ovulate and when we can take a home pregnancy test. Two weeks might as well be next year when all we can think about is seeing that blessed plus sign.

For me, the two-week wait brings a mixture of excited wonder and extended worry. I become consumed by the what-ifs and the what-if-it's-not.

Honestly, both possibilities make me sweat. Either I'm not pregnant, which would crush me, yet again. Or I'm pregnant and could lose the baby, yet again. Pain seems to win no matter what.

Every month, we wrestle with not knowing if or how we'll be devastated. And because we can't control our potential devastation, we let fear take hold and spin us into chaos.

Two-Week Tornado

Take a deep breath, sister. The two-week panic is all too real. When you combine swirling questions with surging hormones, it's understandable that you'd feel overwhelmed. A counselor once told me, "Kelley, don't rush to the next thing or feeling. Deal with the one before you so you'll be ready for the next."

Is there a bigger concern or fear that brings you the most anxiety? Start there. It could be having another miscarriage, having to wait longer, wondering if you're doing something wrong, or the unknown of whether or not you'll ever have a child. The feelings we dwell on can become the things we believe, and the things we believe determine our hearts' direction.

Instead of letting your emotions take your thoughts captive, look to the God of the universe who created you, the world, and everything in it. Colossians 1:17 says, "He is before all things, and in him all things hold together." That includes you. He's holding *you* together. Nothing—including the heartache of infertility—is out of his control.

While it's difficult not knowing his plans or timeline, you can be encouraged that God remembers you and cares deeply about you. The psalmist said, "Your eyes saw me when I was formless; all my days were written in your book and planned before a single one of them began" (Psalm 139:16 csb).

Calm Your Mind Storm

During the two-week wait you've probably wondered if hope is a lost cause. Maybe you can relate to how my friend Jaclyn felt after years of trying to conceive: "Hope was making a fool out of me."

I've also heard people say, "I'm cautiously optimistic," and I've tried it myself. These two contradictory words mean guardedly positive or carefully confident. And yet we aren't actually confident because we're careful. Nor are we truly positive because we're guarded. During an impossibly complex season of infertility, these are valid attempts at self-protection, a tool our brains use to combat our fears.

By trying not to hope, we buy into a false peace. This peace is a controlled variable in our experiment. In reality we're still grasping to control the outcome and manage how much we'll hurt in the end. To calm the mind storm, we need to give our fears over to the one who brings true peace.

Paul told the church at Corinth to "take captive every thought to make it obedient to Christ" (2 Corinthians 10:5). The Message version of this verse offers a rich word picture: "We use our powerful God-tools for smashing warped philosophies, tearing down barriers erected against the truth of God, *fitting every loose thought and emotion and impulse into the structure of life shaped by Christ.* Our tools are ready at hand for clearing the ground of every obstruction and building lives of obedience into maturity" (vv. 5–6, emphasis added).

When you hand over your worries to Christ, you tear down every twisted belief that formed as you've been trying to survive infertility. Once you make this powerful mental shift, the two-week wait becomes less consuming. Your mind is set free, and you can start to see hope in a different light.

Peacefulness Is Provided

In John 14:27, Jesus made an amazing statement: "Peace I leave with you; my peace I give you. I do not give to you as the world gives. Do not let your hearts be troubled and do not be afraid." Only Jesus provides supernatural peace. He's the reason we don't have to be cautiously optimistic. His peace isn't gone tomorrow or in two weeks. No, it outlasts whatever situation we're in.

Fear doesn't own you. Set your mind on Christ's victorious power. He can carry you through the two-week wait and your entire infertility journey. Trust the one who promises, *I will be with you.*

Reflect

- What are your fears on this journey? Be specific. Are you afraid of a certain diagnosis, fertility treatments, having another miscarriage, not ever getting pregnant?

_____

_____

_____

_____

_____

- Do you believe it's possible to be "anxious for nothing" (Philippians 4:6 NKJV)? Why or why not?

_____

_____

_____

_____

_____

- Do you feel cautiously optimistic about your wait? If so, how would you like your mindset to be different?

_____

_____

_____

_____

_____

Pray

Lord, your Word says I can cast all my worries on you because you care for and sustain me (1 Peter 5:7). Yes, Lord, I need you in every minute of my two-week wait. You've promised to be with me, so please help me remember you are here. Your nearness brings trust that helps me develop peace in my waiting instead *of being consumed with fear in the unknown. Protect my mind from all the what-ifs racing through my thoughts and creating anxiety instead of allowing me to focus on wisdom and truth. Keep my mind on what is true. Help me not to overanalyze every detail as I desperately hope this month is it. Help me trust and pray knowing that you can do it, but that even if you do not, you are still trustworthy regardless of the outcome.*

Act

When you start to feel anxious, overwhelmed, or unsteady, try this breathing exercise. Inhale as you name your fears (for example, "This cycle didn't work and I might never get pregnant"). Then exhale slowly as you remind yourself of truths about Jesus (for example, "Jesus is holding me," or "Jesus gives me peace"). The two-week tornado doesn't have to unsettle your mind. Instead, you can take every thought captive and cover it with truth.

Are you having shortness of breath, heart palpitations, changes in sleeping, constant worry, extreme irritability and frustration, or the inability to concentrate on anything other than infertility? If so, you might be experiencing clinical anxiety, says therapist and Waiting in Hope adviser Cathie Quillet. She recommends finding a counselor who specializes in reproductive mental health. Anxiety during infertility leads to anxiety later in life and during pregnancy, as well as postpartum anxiety, she says. Better to address it as soon as you notice symptoms.

Who Am I, If Not a Mother?

See what great love the Father has lavished on us,
that we should be called children of God!

1 John 3:1

My biological clock started ticking in kindergarten. It wasn't that I (Jenn) was boy crazy. For all I understood or cared about at that point in life, a boy wasn't a necessary part of the equation to have a baby.

Through a combination of natural instinct and getting to job-shadow my own incredible mother, the desire to be a mom bloomed in me before I learned how to tie my shoes. I spent hours rocking my Cabbage Patch dolls; pretending to nurse my stuffed rabbit, Trix; and lecturing the neighbor kids about washing their hands and remembering to say please and thank you. Ask my younger sister and brother, and they'll tell you how much I mothered them, along with every small pet or human within arm's reach.

Does my childhood sound like yours? For many of us, the maternal drive kicks in when we're basically babies ourselves. I wasn't the only girl in kindergarten who responded to the question, "What do you want to be when you grow up?" with, "A mom!"

However, you might have a story similar to my friend Brittany's.

Becoming a mom wasn't something she thought about or looked forward to until she and her husband started trying to get pregnant. Then she went through multiple miscarriages, and her heart changed. "Losing babies is really what caused me to want babies," she said. "The Lord grew my desire for children and made me want to live out my motherhood."

In my case, when my husband and I couldn't get pregnant after years of trying, it seemed like someone had ripped my purpose out from under me. Though I worked full-time as an editor, raising babies was my ultimate career goal. As infertility threatened to destroy my beautiful plans, I wondered about the future—what I'd do with my life, where I'd channel my nurturing energy, how I'd ever be happy if I didn't fulfill my calling.

If I wasn't a mother, who was I?

A Relational Lens

If you're feeling lost, confused, or full of self-doubt, know you're not alone. Facing a life crisis like miscarriage and infertility would throw any woman into an identity crisis.

Be encouraged by the truth that who we are is defined by Who made us. And who God says we are remains the same regardless of our motherhood status.

Of all the identities we try on, the most authentic is our identity as God's children. The Bible tells us he adopted us into his family through the Holy Spirit. Unlike other labels we give ourselves, "child of God" isn't a rank we can earn or a title we could lose. It's a right the Lord gives to everyone who accepts and believes in Jesus (John 1:12).

Viewing yourself through the lens of your relationship with God can help you work through identity questions that come up during your wait for a child. You're not just a woman who's not yet a mom. You're a daughter of the Most High. As the King's daughter, you're guaranteed divine royalties: sacred affection, eternal protection, limitless grace, and the honor of calling him "Abba," which means "Daddy" (Romans 8:15).

Thinking of God as your father might be difficult. It's a sad reality that many children grow up with a dad who abused them, abandoned the family, or wasn't involved in parenting. If daddy imagery is tough for you, picture the most caring older man you know, maybe a pastor, Sunday school teacher, or neighbor. Think of how he treats his family with tenderness and tries to keep them safe. This is just a beginning to help you see God for who he is—except your heavenly Father never loses his temper, always keeps his promises, and understands your heart better than you do.

God knows that everything within you is screaming, "I was meant to be a mom!" In your mourning for dreams that haven't come true, he will comfort you with love that is sure.

Career Versus Identity

A few weeks before I wrote this chapter, United States gymnast Simone Biles shocked the world when she withdrew from competition during the women's team final at the 2020 Olympic Games (which were held in 2021). Simone, who's unquestionably one of the greatest gymnasts of all time, later explained she wasn't feeling mentally able to continue and didn't want to risk injury or cost her team a medal.

Although many people criticized the superstar gymnast, others praised her decision to protect her mental health. In response to the positive feedback, she tweeted, "the outpouring [of] love & support I've received has made me realize I'm more than my accomplishments and gymnastics which I never truly believed before."[1]

I may not have seven Olympic medals to my name, but I can relate to how Simone tied her identity to her career. I've done the same thing with motherhood.

During my struggle with infertility, I saw myself as a loser. I latched on to the idea that being a mom was what a woman was supposed to be. After all, God gave us the physical tools to grow life. Because I wasn't performing the job I was made for, I felt worthless. It took me years to realize I was only making myself unhappy measuring who I was by what I couldn't produce.

Like Simone, we're more than what we do or, in this season of waiting, what we *want* to do.

Motherhood is a worthy and desirable role, but it's not the center of a woman's life. It can't be. No occupation can anchor our identity. Basing our sense of self on external things—our jobs, achievements, social status, marriage, and other relationships—sets us up for disappointment. The minute something or someone fails to meet our expectations, our stability crumbles.

Friend, hear me out. There's nothing wrong with wanting to be a mom. You're longing to fulfill a vital calling. But think about the little hands you wish to clasp—they're simply not strong enough to carry such a weighty responsibility as defining your identity.

As we saw in chapter 1, God created us "in his own image" (Genesis 1:27). This is why all human life holds immeasurable value. Every person reflects different aspects of our Maker. Our lives matter, not because of what we accomplish but because we're God's accomplishment.

Ephesians 2:10 describes how God created us for his purposes to carry out his plans. I encourage you to personalize the message and meditate on its significance: "For [I am] God's handiwork, created in Christ Jesus to do good works, which God prepared in advance for [me] to do."

Through whatever work you do, even as you're waiting to become a mom, you can display the beauty of your Creator.

Who You Truly Are

If I could travel back a couple of decades and give my frizzy-banged, buck-toothed kindergarten self a word of advice, I know what I'd say:

Little Jenn, go ahead and dream of being a mom. Keep strolling your stuffed dog around the living room and whispering bedtime prayers over your toy ponies. You're dabbling in the art of motherly love, a form of sacrifice that brings joy to your heart and glory to God.

Also, know this: motherhood isn't your identity. Your life won't transform from meaningless to purposeful once you welcome a child into your arms. The core of who you are lies deeper than any earthly label you hope to gain.

Just as Jesus called the bleeding woman who clutched at his robe (Matthew 9:22), God has named you "Daughter." You belong to him. The things of this world—even good things like being a mom—shift and fade over time, but your heavenly Father's care for you will last, forever and always. So look to him and believe your worth.

This applies to you too. If you know Jesus, you're God's beloved child. He made you, chose you, and draped you in his radiance.

Be confident in Christ as you walk through this identity crisis. The Spirit will lead you, because you are his. "I am convinced and confident of this very thing, that He who has begun a good work in you will [continue to] perfect and complete it until the day of Christ Jesus [the time of His return]" (Philippians 1:6 AMP).

Reflect

- How do you see yourself right now? Are you focusing more on what you want to be—a mother—or on what you have through Christ—a relationship with God as his daughter?

_____

_____

_____

_____

- In his book *Abba's Child*, author Brennan Manning encourages followers of Jesus to "define yourself radically as one beloved by God."[2] Would you define yourself this way, or does that make you uncomfortable? If the picture of God as your Father brings up difficult memories, write what you feel. Then ask the Lord to help you see him clearly, convinced that he's far better than any earthly father.

_____

_____

_____

_____

_____

- Do you feel like your life is on hold or purposeless? Answer honestly, and consider whether you might be attaching your identity to the work of motherhood.

_____

_____

_____

_____

_____

Pray

My Father, it's hard not to feel like my life is falling apart. With infertility putting motherhood seemingly out of reach, I'm struggling to know who I am. I need you to shine your truth into my confusion. Let the reassurance of being your child comfort my ache over not being a mother or over missing my baby (or babies) in heaven. Thank you for creating me as a portrait of your majesty. Help me step into the roles and life work where you place me so I can share how amazing it is to be loved by you.

Act

In the journaling space here, from memory or using a Bible search tool, write biblical declarations of who God says you are. For example, "I am chosen," "I am holy in God's sight," and "I am beloved" (see Ephesians 1:4). Then, copy the declarations onto sticky notes and post them on your bathroom mirror. Read the declarations out loud in the morning to start your day with truth.

4

Sighs of Sorrow

Be merciful to me, Lord, for I am in distress; my eyes
grow weak with sorrow, my soul and body with grief.

Psalm 31:9

Empty. Utterly empty. That's all I (Kelley) felt. Emptiness and disbelief. I pushed up off the bathroom floor, careful not to slide on the puddle of tears. My clothes were still damp from when this nightmare began. Overcome by pain, I was exhausted beyond anything I'd ever known. An hour had passed, maybe more. I couldn't fathom what my body had just determined without my say-so. Staring at the tile and holes in the grout, I felt as close as I could get to death. Death was inside me.

Time seemed to be moving backward in those minutes and days after my second miscarriage. I knew deep within me the moment the cramping and bleeding began that things were *not* okay. I had already been through an early miscarriage, which happened more quickly than I expected. Since seeing the blood clot in the toilet, I hadn't had time to process what had happened or what I'd lost.

Now, with my third miscarriage, I knew what the next few days would hold. At our ten-week checkup, the eerie silence during the sonogram made my heart sink. The doctor confirmed what I dreaded. "I'm sorry; there is no longer a heartbeat. Your baby probably stopped growing at eight weeks." My body was clearly in disbelief, and so was my mind.

My future changed again in an instant. My heart was broken yet again.

Infertility Is Grief

Those of us who struggle with infertility are no strangers to loss. Miscarriage, ectopic pregnancy, stillbirth, and fatal diagnoses are often our reality.

Whether or not our story includes miscarriage, we all suffer crushed expectations and missed opportunities to experience motherhood. Growing our family looks different from what we'd hoped. We had ideas for surprising our husbands or getting pregnant at the same time as a friend, but our plans fell to pieces. Even our menstrual cycles represent loss. A friend of mine calls her period a "monthly funeral for my dreams."

Infertility is more than just grief; infertility is trauma. Defined as a traumatic experience, reproductive trauma is "the stressors of infertility (and all other reproductive events) [that] occur in existential, physical, emotional, and interpersonal realms and may be beyond the average person's coping abilities."[1]

As we try to cope, it can be tempting to minimize our grief. We internalize comments like, "At least it's not cancer," and then beat ourselves up for feeling sad. Or we hear impersonal words uttered at the doctor's office and start to doubt. *Did I go through a biological process called "pregnancy loss"—or did I lose a person growing in my womb?*

Instead of downplaying grief, we can take comfort knowing God validates our losses. The story of Hannah shows that not being able to conceive causes great anguish (1 Samuel 1:16). God's Word also upholds the sanctity of life, the belief that life begins at the earliest moment when sperm meets egg. (Biblical references to human life in the womb include Psalm 139:13–16, Jeremiah 1:5, and Luke 1:41–44.)

Dear one, this means that your early miscarriage was a baby. The little one you delivered without breath in her lungs was a baby. The embryo you transferred to your womb was a baby. These are all lives worthy of grief. All your losses of infertility are worth grieving.

God knows how much you're hurting. You can go to him when the grief of your wait feels stifling. It's okay to tell him that you're not okay.

Even Jesus Wept

When sorrow presses on us like a dark cloud, how do we find the strength to make it through each painful day? We look to God's Word for examples of his faithfulness, his safety in hard times, his help when we cry out in our distress, and his nearness.

In Psalm 31, David spoke honestly with God. He reminded himself that God heard his cries. Even better, God did not just listen to David's cries; he cared. In the same way, God actively carries us in the middle of our sorrow.

- Turn your ear to me, come quickly to my rescue; be my rock of refuge, a strong fortress to save me. (v. 2)
- Into your hands I commit my spirit; deliver me, LORD, my faithful God. (v. 5)
- Be merciful to me, LORD, for I am in distress; my eyes grow weak with sorrow, my soul and body with grief. My life is consumed by anguish and my years by groaning; my strength fails because of my affliction, and my bones grow weak. (vv. 9–10)

- But I trust in you, LORD; I say, "You are my God." My times are in your hands. (vv. 14–15)
- In my alarm I said, "I am cut off from your sight!" Yet you heard my cry for mercy when I called to you for help. (v. 22)

During my miscarriages, I could hear the echoes of God's love. As I poured out my heart to him, I lamented (cried out) for help and strength like David. I pleaded with God to show me his nearness and hold me tighter than the cold bathroom floor's embrace. In my rawness, I saw the Lord God who cries with us.

Can you picture that? God crying with you as you mourn the losses of infertility? I know it can be hard, depending on where you're at in your faith or if you wouldn't call yourself a Christian.

There's a story in the Bible that can help us believe what we can't visualize. Mary and Martha were grieving the death of their brother, Lazarus. The Gospel of John tells us that when Jesus saw the sisters weeping, "he was deeply moved in spirit and troubled" (11:33). But there's more. He didn't just feel bad and take pity on them. "Jesus wept" (v. 35).

Here we see the deep and intimate love Christ has for us. The Son of God, clothed in human flesh, demonstrated how he lets us run to him and release our tears.

Weeping is so crucial that Jesus had to show us how it's done. Instead of instantly healing Lazarus or quickly moving on, Jesus wept. In his crying with us, we find lasting comfort.

Soothe Your Mourning Heart

Believe that grief will not overcome you. When you feel like you'll succumb to the pain, God will hold you together. He does not leave us to sigh alone.

"You have collected all my tears and preserved them in your bottle! You have recorded every one in your book" (Psalm 56:8 TLB).

You can't rush past the aches that linger deep within you. Your loss is not forgotten. Your babies matter. They'll always remain in your heart and in God's care.

Thankfully, our Savior redeems the pain as he touches our wounds and applies his healing balm. However, this new skin looks different. It's a reminder of his work in our hearts. I've seen God take the desolation of loss and bring beauty from my ashes, as only his tender hand can do. The Lord's compassionate love for you will soothe your mourning heart if you let him.

Reflect

- What has caused you grief in your journey thus far? How does it make you feel to learn that infertility is trauma?

_____

_____

_____

_____

_____

_____

_____

_____

- Have you taken the time to grieve your losses of infertility and miscarriage (if applicable)? Why or why not?

_____

_____

_____

_____

_____

- How have you shared your grief with others? If you haven't, what step will you take to share your grief with someone?

_____

_____

_____

_____

_____

_____

Pray

Lord, please be merciful to me; I need you. Like David, I'm crying out to you for help. I'm weary from grief and weak with sorrow. No one can ease this pain but you, God. Help me trust you more, even when the pain is deep and doesn't make sense. Thank you for reminding me that you care intimately about my sorrow, and you store my tears. Come quickly to heal these open wounds of my heart. Lord, hold me; put me back together with your healing hands. In you, I commit my heart and my spirit.

Act

If you have lost a baby through miscarriage or stillbirth, consider memorializing your baby with a gift, book, tree, or yearly reminder of this life that matters. If your journey doesn't include infant loss, consider journaling and discussing with someone your feelings on the grief and trauma of infertility.

See a licensed professional counselor if you feel heavy from grief and the cloud of depression and sorrow isn't lifting, especially if you're feeling hopeless. Don't walk through the loss alone; grief can heal in community.

5

Freedom from Shame

Because the Sovereign LORD helps me, I will not be disgraced. Therefore have I set my face like flint, and I know I will not be put to shame.

Isaiah 50:7

I'm broken.
I waited too long to get married and start a family.
God must not be giving me a baby because I'd be a bad mom.
It's my fault.

Enter the mind games of infertility. This painful time of not getting pregnant and losing babies opens us up to the lies of shame. Perhaps you've felt embarrassed, inferior, or less-than because of your fertility struggles. I (Jenn) did more times than I could count. When waiting at the gynecologist's office, I'd look at the women cradling their baby bumps and say to myself, *You don't belong here.* The same lie hounded me at church. I braved going one Mother's Day Sunday and immediately regretted it. You can only take so much humiliation watching other women stand for applause while you—the odd woman out—have to stay in your seat.

Shame is specific in its accusations. You might feel ashamed that your body isn't working right, that you haven't exhausted all your options to try to get pregnant, or that you can't make your husband a dad. If you had a miscarriage, you might think you didn't take care of your body enough to keep your baby safe and healthy. Secondary infertility can also bring about feelings of shame that you're not thankful for the child you have or that you're a bad parent for not giving your child a sibling.

My friend Kayla battled shame about her diet and health choices. After being diagnosed with polycystic ovary syndrome (PCOS), she became consumed with finding out how to correct her hormonal imbalances and get pregnant naturally.

"I thought if I could eat the right foods, exercise more, take the right supplements, or figure out the actual root cause I would at least know I did everything I could," she said.

Determined not to go through medical treatments, Kayla tried different natural remedies without success. She went back and forth between wanting to give up and working harder to find a solution. The burden of trying to fix herself wore her down emotionally and spiritually.

She shared, "I felt like I was letting God down and myself down."

Shame's Beginning

Like Kayla, many of us have to fight the belief that we're a failure if we can't conceive or carry a baby. Infertility is so humiliating that we can start to hate our bodies and feel like everything we do is wrong.

Where does shame come from? And why is it so hard to get rid of? God's Word explains that we inherited shame from our oldest ancestors. When Adam and Eve ate the fruit God commanded them not to eat in the garden of Eden, they suddenly realized they were naked. Up until then, wearing clothes wasn't a thing. The first man and woman didn't worry about being exposed because they had nothing to hide.

However, as soon as they sinned, Adam and Eve felt the urge to cover themselves. Adam told God why: "I heard you in the garden, and I was afraid because I was naked; so I hid" (Genesis 3:10). And so shame was born. Disobedience against God brought disgrace before him.

Not only did Adam and Eve ruin their standing with the Lord, but they also wrecked life for the rest of us. Through what's called the fall, the world became stained by sin. The act of breaking God's law ushered pain and death into creation. We all suffer from the aftermath of the first sin and add our own sins to the earth's troubles.

I realize that going over the effects of sin sounds like a lousy pep talk. But let me tell you how our ancient backstory can offer us comfort. Shame and infertility share the same birthday. Eve's sin brought a specific consequence for her and for us: "pains in childbearing" (Genesis 3:16). Everything hard about the reproductive process—heavy periods, PMS, miscarriage, ovulation problems, labor, and delivery—can be traced to the fall. Sin's mark on us as women includes female health issues that, for the most part, we can't control. This is also true for male factor infertility and medical problems in general.

Hear this truth: *infertility isn't your fault.* The shame you feel comes from the consequences of sin affecting your or your husband's biology. You and I *are* broken as we suffer the effects of the fall. Yet God has provided a way to make us whole without the burden of shame.

The Perfect Remedy

While we can take steps to treat the medical causes of infertility, we're ultimately not in charge of when, how, or if we'll get pregnant or have children by other means. That fact can both give us relief and make us uncomfortable.

In his book *Shame Interrupted*, psychologist Ed Welch talked about how shame can be especially tempting when we feel powerless: "Perhaps we blame ourselves because in a strange way it helps us feel as though we have more control. If we are responsible for whatever went wrong, for whatever hurt us, we might be able to figure out how to keep it from happening again."[1] This is how shame latches on during our waiting journey. We sense an urgency to take back control and stop the pain from breaking us. But unfortunately, our attempts to control our circumstances are about as effective as Adam and Eve's leafy rags. They're a Band-Aid on a deep wound. What we need is a lasting remedy that cures the source of all that hurts us.

God sent his Son for this exact purpose. Second Corinthians 5:21 says, "God made him who had no sin to be sin for us, so that in him we might become the righteousness of God." Jesus took our sin and gave us his perfection. Instead of death, we get new life. His sacrifice guarantees that every wrong we do and every wrong done to us will one day be made right.

Do you believe that? In Jesus, you're blameless. Your sins are forgiven; your relationship with God is secured. He has made you a new creation, no longer exposed and afraid of the future. You don't have to try to protect yourself, because God has set you apart for his purposes—purposes that are good and kind and give honor to him. So trust that his Word is true and that shame is a liar.

Holy and Free

After God called out Adam and Eve for their disobedience, he dressed them in animal skins. They needed him to cover their shame. Through Jesus, God offers us complete covering—his own holiness.

While the world's brokenness still brings us sorrow and shame, we know these are temporary problems. Death was beaten. In the end, Jesus wins. As Isaiah said, "He will swallow up death forever. The Sovereign LORD will wipe away the tears from all faces; he will remove his people's disgrace from all the earth" (Isaiah 25:8).

I hope those words lift the weight off your shoulders. You don't have to own the shame of infertility. It's not your burden to carry. Let the truth of your new life in Christ free you from the mind games. You can wait unashamed under the protection of your Savior.

Reflect

- How have you felt shame during your wait for a child?

_____

_____

_____

_____

_____

- Do you feel the instinct to run or hide if someone knows you're going through infertility? If so, why?

_____

_____

_____

_____

_____

- Ed Welch wrote, "Shame will never surrender its power over you if you are tentative about it. You need to identify it and attack it with hope."[2] How can hope in Jesus help you fight shame?

_____

_____

_____

_____

_____

_____

Pray

Dear Jesus, after trying for so long and not getting pregnant, I can't help but think I did something wrong. I keep having thoughts that I could have stopped infertility from happening and that I should do more to fix it. I'm ashamed that my body is failing at growing a baby. Help me remember that infertility was caused by the fall. I need your grace to accept the freedom you bought for me. Renew my mind to focus on your holiness that covers my sin and shame.

Act

Get some paper and draw three columns. In the first column, note which lies of shame you keep hearing. In the second, say how the lie makes you feel. In the third, write what God's Word says to counter the lie. You can find verses about specific topics by doing a keyword search at a website such as blueletterbible.org or using a Bible app on your phone.

Shame can follow difficult and traumatic circumstances such as sexual sin, abortion, and physical or emotional abuse. If your shame feels deep and irrevocable, please seek Christian counseling and other mental health care. The Lord can help you find healing and forgiveness to break these heavy chains.

6

Too Weak to Carry On

But he said to me, "My grace is sufficient for you,
for my power is made perfect in weakness."

2 Corinthians 12:9

I (Kelley) had been through a few wild months as every fluid ounce of my body had been checked at the fertility clinic. Yet they still needed a hysteroscopy to confirm that my tubes and uterus were clear.

My husband, Justin, couldn't take off for another appointment, so I asked my friend Becky to take me. Once at the surgery center, she worked to calm my nerves. My open gown provided plenty of giggly distractions. If only that had been the funniest thing of that day. I placed my loose clothing into the personal items bag before they began my IV. After that, everything was a blur.

Becky later told me that I struggled to wake from anesthesia. However, instead of allowing me time to recover, the nurses told her to get me dressed to go. I'm not sure why they didn't let me recover, but I wish they had. Becky proceeded to describe how she put my thong underwear back on me.

Yes, I chose the most embarrassing day to wear my skimpiest undies. Continuing the ridiculousness of the moment, I began yelling, "My clothes are attacking me!" as she wheeled me out. Even though this is now a hilarious joke in our bonded friendship, that day's bareness (literally) depicts the weakness I felt.

Keeping a sense of humor can be a helpful coping strategy. But most of the time, the weariness of infertility is anything but funny.

We endure much from the discomfort of fertility tests, treatments, surgeries, and constantly changing procedures or medications. Not to mention the unexpected diagnosis of a chronic illness that explains some of the weird things happening to our bodies, yet at the same time leaves us completely confused.

For example, PCOS and endometriosis cause pain and issues like ovarian cysts, migraines, severe cramps, and fatigue. PCOS is the most common cause of female infertility, affecting about five million women of childbearing age in the United States.[1] Endometriosis affects more than 176 million women worldwide, though that number might be higher because the disease is often misdiagnosed.[2]

If you suffer from reproductive health issues, you know how exhausting they can be. It doesn't take long before you experience the complex, uncomfortable, and shocking moments that make you weary when you're waiting for a child.

Hitting the Wall

Walking through infertility takes a toll not only on your heart but also on your body. The repetitive discomfort of poking, probing, pills, and pain can easily lead you to an exhausted, sore, and sick state.

I remember one moment when I looked at Justin with tears streaming down my pale face. I whimpered, "I can't. I need a break." My white flag waved. It was God's grace to give me this perspective. I was beyond weary; the all-consuming infertility battle took me as its prisoner. You may be thinking, *Kelley, aren't you being dramatic?* Yes, but honestly, I had hit a wall. The grief, testing, surgeries, and failed attempts had taken their toll, and I couldn't do it anymore.

I had nothing to offer in my complete weakness. But I could be honest with God. I could show him my raw self. Thankfully, the Lord loves to meet us when and where life hurts.

Looking through the Bible, you'll see many weak and weary hearts that needed rescue. Each person reached a point of being physically weak, tired, and in pain. Even Jesus, who for our sake set aside his power and glory to walk the earth like us, needed a break. He was tempted in the desert and had deep bodily aches; he had to escape the crowds; and even in the garden of Gethsemane, Jesus experienced grave agony.

We understand David's plea in Psalm 6:2: "Have mercy on me and be gracious to me, O Lord, for I am weak (faint, frail); Heal me, O Lord, for my bones are dismayed and anguished" (AMP). God knows our pain and does not want us to struggle alone in silence. Verse 9 confirms what we yearn to hear: "The Lord has heard my supplication [my plea for grace]; The Lord receives my prayer" (AMP).

We sometimes forget that God does not force himself, his power, or his authority on us. No, just the opposite. In his unfailing, steadfast love and mercy (v. 4), we see he can save us and rescue our souls. If we allow him to work in our weakness, we will have great strength at our fingertips. Can you believe we have access to the power of the Creator, Savior, Redeemer, and God Almighty, who has already conquered the grave, forever?

We're all either heading into a storm, going through a storm, or coming out of a storm in life. We can't avoid pain in a broken world, but we're safer with God as our protector.

God's Strength, Not Ours

Maybe during hard times you've heard someone say, "God won't give you more than you can handle." Though it's an attempt to make you feel better, this statement with good intentions falls short. Not only that, but this phrase is *not* a Bible verse or biblical truth.

I entered infertility already acquainted with suffering after decades of chronic pain, which we learned in 2019 was from a rare brain disorder I was born with. Chiari malformation had debilitating effects on my life that snowballed into my infertility. During these times of weakness, I clung to the Amplified translation of 2 Corinthians 12:9:

> But He has said to me, "My grace is sufficient for you [My lovingkindness and My mercy are more than enough—always available—regardless of the situation]; for [My] power is being perfected [and is completed and shows itself most effectively] in [your] weakness." Therefore, I will all the more gladly boast in my weaknesses, so that the power of Christ [may completely enfold me and] may dwell in me.

Christ's supernatural power shows itself most effective in your human weakness. I learned this firsthand as the pain compounded and I grew empty—yet the Lord's grace covered me. Like David in Psalm 6, my desperate need for God brought me into God's strong and mighty hands in my pleading and incapability. Remember, he won't push his way in. Just as in any good relationship, intimacy is not created by force. Our hearts' pleas ask him to draw nearer.

Today admitting weakness seems countercultural, even in the Christian women's sphere. We're being told, "You're a warrior!" This is misguided theology. Instead, the Bible says we are all humans—frail and in need. Peter said in 1 Peter 1:24–25, "All people are like grass, and all their glory is like the flowers of the field; the grass withers and the flowers fall, but the word of the Lord endures forever." And Paul said in Acts 17:28 that it's only because of Christ in us that we live and breathe and can do anything.

God *does* allow us to walk through more than we can handle *on our own*. When we are at the end of ourselves, we can rely on God's power, not our efforts. He wants us to realize our need for him.

He not only joins us in our suffering here and now, but he rescues us forever. Therefore, we can believe and rest in the beautiful resolution that Jesus has ultimate victory over the final wall in our weakness: death.

Let Weariness Take You Deeper

Infertility reveals that you can't help yourself. You cannot change your circumstance no matter how hard you try.

I encourage you to let the struggles of infertility lead you to a deeper, not weaker, place. Only God gives us endurance, but we must ask for it and rely on him. Our efforts will fail every time in any hard place.

In this exhausting journey, we can trust the one who has all power, authority, and might. Our God will never grow weary. It's in him alone that we can be strong. So when you find yourself at a brick wall, unable to keep going, you can gain all of his never-ending strength to carry on.

Reflect

- In what ways have you felt weak and weary from your journey? Tell God where you're hitting the wall.

_____

_____

_____

_____

_____

- What does God's Word say about your weaknesses in 2 Corinthians
  12:9? It's helpful to compare different versions such as Amplified and
  The Message in your observation.

_____

_____

_____

_____

_____

- How can you find strength in the Lord instead of yourself?

_____

_____

_____

_____

_____

Pray

Dear Lord, you know the weariness and pain I'm feeling and how weak it's made me. Will you give me strength through the power of the Holy Spirit? Psalm 46 says you are my refuge and strength, my helper who is always found in times of trouble. May I believe you are my Lord who fights for me; I need only to be still. Give me strength in your name to make it through the next step you lead me to.

Act

When we're too weak to carry on, we need to ask for help. Tonight, share with your husband how you're feeling and suggest a way he could help relieve some of the heaviness. Also, plan to reach out to one other person you can ask to help you walk through this journey. Even Moses needed other people to hold up his arms when he got too tired (Exodus 17:11–13).

7

Why Her and Not Me?

A heart at peace gives life to the body, but envy rots the bones.

Proverbs 14:30

The call came while we were eating dinner. My husband, Colin, answered as I (Jenn) twirled more strands of pad thai around my fork. One look at his shocked and then pained expression, and I knew immediately: it was bad news.

It turned out I was wrong. The news was wonderful—just hard to hear. Colin's brother called to let us know he and his wife, Kim, were pregnant. Barely six months into their marriage, they were already expecting. Meanwhile, Colin and I had six *years* of marriage under our belts with no children to show for it. In a twist of cruel timing, we had just learned our IVF cycle had to be postponed due to a cyst found on one of my ovaries.

As soon as my husband uttered the words "Kim is pregnant," an invisible fist slammed into me. Heat rose in my throat, but not because of the spice. The grief I'd tried to ignore rushed to the surface, heaving in a burst of tears.

Does this experience hit home for you? Odds are, you've been in my position before—the victim of a pregnancy announcement gut punch. One minute, you're calmly scrolling through social media—and then *bam*! You see a sonogram image or a dog with a "Big Sister" sign on its neck, and your day is ruined.

Most of the time, you're genuinely happy for the other person. For example, I was thrilled my in-laws were pregnant and looked forward to being Aunt Jenn. It's not that you don't want *her* to have a baby. You want *both* of you to have babies.

But then there are times we despise the pregnant woman. The teen mom, the meth addict, the housewife with half a dozen kids. We don't want *her* to have a baby because we think she doesn't deserve one.

Whether or not we feel happy for the woman who's expecting, we can't avoid the difference between us. She has what our hearts ache for. Sadly, trying to stifle the pain and paste on a smile only works for so long.

It's hard to say congrats when we're choking back sobs.

From Injury to Envy

You and I feel this struggle often. On a good day, we might be able to name what we're battling besides infertility: that green-eyed monster, envy. As Proverbs 14:30 says, "A peaceful heart leads to a healthy body; jealousy is like cancer in the bones" (NLT). If comparison is the thief of joy, then envy is the destroyer of peace. It blames other people for the unfairness of life, making us sick with spite.

The sneaky thing about envy is that it starts as harmless. We have a desire for something good—a promotion, a bigger house, a baby. The desire itself isn't sinful. But not getting what we desire hurts. And seeing someone else get what we so desperately want adds insult to injury. In my opinion, this is one of the worst side effects of infertility. One woman's joy triggers another's sorrow.

When the shock of a pregnancy announcement wears off, and we're raw with grief, our hearts beg God for an explanation. *Why did you give her a baby, but not me?*

This question signals the turning point in the progression of envy. After that, we either release the hurt to Jesus or bury it as resentment. If we choose to bury it, resentment then grows into bitterness, which damages our relationship with the other person and ultimately makes us even more miserable than we were in the first place.

Our Model for Heartache

I don't have to tell you envy is wrong. You probably feel guilty already and wish you could quit caring about other women's pregnancies.

But let's be real. We can't snap our fingers and make our emotions disappear. Thankfully, God's Word gives us an example of how to process our grief without sinning.

The first chapter of 1 Samuel tells the story of Hannah, a childless Jewish woman married to a man named Elkanah. Hannah not only faced the shame of being barren in a culture that prized fertility, but she was also mocked by her husband's other wife, Peninnah, who had a whole pack of sons and daughters.

Year after year, Elkanah gathered his family and traveled to make sacrifices at the temple. Every time they made the trip, Peninnah teased Hannah mercilessly for her lack of children. Imagine how agonizing that would be, having your heartache rubbed in your face.

We wouldn't fault Hannah if she had envied Peninnah, especially after all the torment Peninnah caused. But envy wasn't Hannah's response.

Instead of taking out her frustration on her rival, Hannah took her sorrow to the Lord. There at the temple, unconcerned about the mess she must have looked like to anyone watching, Hannah prayed and wept and poured out her soul. She believed that God was listening and trusted that he would care for what and who was troubling her.

Guide Your Emotions

Hannah's example shows us that avoiding envy is possible. To help steer your emotions in the right direction, be intentional and ACT:

- *Acknowledge* your grief. Take time to journal, chat with a friend, and/or see a counselor.
- *Confess* if you've been allowing envy to grow. And if the pregnant woman you envy sinned against you, forgive her.
- *Thank* God for the new life he creates, the comfort he provides, and the forgiveness he extends to his struggling children.

The Lord knows your anguish after a pregnancy announcement gut punch. The jumble of emotions you feel doesn't overwhelm him. He can show you how to be both sad for you and glad for her.

Reflect

- How do you usually react to a pregnancy announcement?

_____

_____

_____

_____

_____

- Have you talked to God about your grief triggered by someone else's pregnancy? Or are you bottling up your pain until it fills you with resentment?

_____

_____

_____

_____

- When you think of your friend, sister-in-law, coworker, or another woman who is pregnant, what are your feelings toward her? What would you like your feelings to be?

_____

_____

_____

_____

Pray

Dear Jesus, I know your Word says I should rejoice with those who rejoice and weep with those who weep (Romans 12:15). But hearing another woman rejoice about her pregnancy makes me weep. Even though I'm usually happy for her, I wrestle with envy because she has what I desperately want. I need you to cleanse me from envy's sickness. Forgive me for how I've begrudged her and not trusted your sovereignty over pregnancy. Give me a heart like Hannah's so I can surrender my tears to your tender care.

Act

The next time you hear a pregnancy announcement, follow the "Iris Rule" (named after my friend Iris, who came up with this brilliant idea). From the moment you hear the news, give yourself twenty-four hours to feel every emotion: sadness, anger, confusion, and all the "whys." Write your emotions on a piece of paper. After twenty-four hours, tear up the paper. Next, on a new sheet, write the pregnant woman's name, along with a prayer thanking God for the baby he's forming in her womb and asking for his protection over mother and child. Make praise and prayer your weapons against the temptation of envy.

8

Outside the Mommy Club

Turn to me and be gracious to me, for I am lonely and afflicted.

Psalm 25:16

As the years dragged on, I (Kelley) watched as more and more friends became pregnant and welcomed home babies before me. I never expected to be six years into marriage and still not have a child.

I remember the moment Justin shared another friend's news with me, and I realized we were officially being lapped. Their second birth announcement emphasized the further disappointment I felt for still not joining their club.

This elusive club of motherhood seemed so out of reach. I felt like I was on an island and banned from coming to the mainland that had everything I wanted yet couldn't have.

Saying I was lonely or alone in my aches would be understating the gravity of what I felt. My world reminded me constantly of my lack of club membership. For many years I was inevitably hurt by and excluded from mommy gatherings, baby showers, church moms' groups, and friends' playdates. If I *was* invited, my exclusion quickly followed in the form of dis-connection. I had nothing to offer the conversations regarding mom advice, funny kid stories, or parenting hacks.

The circles I should belong to, I no longer fit into. I felt the pull of our distancing life stages. No matter how hard I tried, the club was out of reach.

Perhaps you are like me, as all I could see were mommy-club members. Everywhere I went, pregnancy bumps, babies, and bouncing toddlers taunted me. They mocked my inability to join their club, and in my mind I further exaggerated just how left out and excluded I was.

You might be like many women in our Waiting in Hope Ministries community who shared, "I'm the only one I know who's going through infertility. Everyone else is pregnant or has kids." Many of us walk this journey not knowing anyone else who shares our struggle. We can further isolate our lonely hearts as we believe the whispers, "You are the only one" and, "You are all alone."

Our viewpoint emphasizes that everyone seems to be moving past us, leaving us out of the only club we yearn to join.

Our Friend in Sorrows

Infertility can create an obvious divide between women: the haves and the have-nots. Our everyday surroundings and encounters reveal this reality. Women—including me and Kayla—who've lost babies are in a third (and confusing) category, the unseen moms who both have and have not.

"The more difficult moments came with basic conversations about birth, breastfeeding, parenting," Kayla said. "Although I had given birth to a stillborn, I didn't feel I could share my experiences in those moments because they would think it was a sad memory. When in reality, I like to share about her birth just like they like to share about their baby's birth."

Similar to Kayla's, my baby mattered. Yet I couldn't speak of my little one, and I didn't have a baby in my arms to verify my mother status.

In such a place, it's hard for our hearts to be present. It's similar to when we hear mommy friends complain about being tired (which I'm sure they are) and say they can't wait for naptime. We sit there quietly, listening yet aching about how we can't wait to hold a baby, even if we're exhausted. There's a sting in hearing them take for granted or struggle in what you and I so desperately want. We try hard not to be angry, but it deeply hurts.

It's normal and completely okay to feel hurt, lonely, and sad from the pain caused by others around you, even though it's probably unintentional. That is acceptable and honestly expected. Seeing that they have children hurts our have-not hearts.

In my lingering self-pity over not feeling as though I fit in with the mommy club, I found Isaiah 53:3: "He was despised and rejected by mankind, a man of suffering, and familiar with pain." Jesus understands us. He was mistreated by many and even abandoned by those closest to him. Jesus is described here as the Man of Sorrows.

The Message version paraphrases Isaiah 53:4 this way: "One look at him and people turned away. We looked down on him, thought he was scum. But the fact is, it was *our* pains he carried—*our* disfigurements, all the things wrong with *us*." The Bible is full of outcasts, lonely and isolated. Jesus knows and carries our hurting hearts.

Never Truly Alone

It's human nature to self-protect, and that is a good response. However, in my infertility loneliness, this coping skill further isolated me when I desperately needed friendships. In my need to be understood and accepted, I allowed the fear of being hurt to cause me to isolate further. Instead of reaching out for help or sharing what I really needed, I caused myself more unnecessary pain.

It's like when I look into my closet and say, "I have nothing to wear." In those moments, my husband, in logical and utter disbelief, says, "Nothing, really?"

I know that's a silly example, but it's true. My feelings and emotions can cloud the reality of what is in front of me. My view causes my heart to become distorted. I start to think, *Friendships are distant or hard right now; therefore, I am all alone.* These emotional and extreme thoughts can take us on a tailspin downward. But truth pulls us in.

Remember God's tenderness and love described in Psalm 34:18? He draws near to the brokenhearted and lost. But he does more than draw near in our pain. He never leaves us. The most beautiful and intimate realization is that you are actually *never* lonely, unseen, or misunderstood.

Psalm 139:7–10 proclaims, "Where can I go from Your Spirit? Or where can I flee from Your presence? If I ascend into heaven, You are there; if I make my bed in hell, behold, You are there. . . . Even there Your hand shall lead me, and Your right hand shall hold me" (NKJV).

We cannot escape God's never-ceasing nearness. No matter what we are feeling or the situation we are in, God is still close. Once we believe the truth that our Father God is with us, we can recognize that the whisper that we are alone is a lie. We were created by God in his image as deeply relational beings.

You are not alone—ever. God is always with you.

Your Shepherd Walks with You

When I looked at the mommy club surrounding me, it was easy to think, *No one understands me.* However, I realized that wasn't true. As I began to share my journey, other women shared theirs. I was *not* the only one—far from it.

We all, as couples, must decide whether to share or not. Chances are there are others around you feeling alone in their journey of infertility too. But even if you've shared and there is still no one who relates, our online community at Waiting in Hope Ministries has thousands who will walk with you.[1]

As I opened up, I experienced unexpected comfort and peace. The deep loneliness and isolation of waiting became easier as I turned to the truth that Jesus is my great, caring Shepherd who is with me. Psalm 23:1–4 says, "The Lord is *my* Shepherd; he leads, refreshes, and guides, and even though I walk through the darkest valley, I will fear no evil, for *you* are walking with *me* and comfort *me*" (my paraphrase).

Reflect

- Describe a time when the words or circumstances of a friend made you feel like a have-not. Do you think the person meant to hurt you? Spend a few minutes writing down your feelings.

_____

_____

_____

_____

_____

_____

- In what ways have you isolated yourself or put up a wall against others?

_____

_____

_____

_____

_____

- Consider the Scriptures used in the chapter, especially Psalm 23. What do you think about Jesus being your Shepherd who walks with you?

_____

_____

_____

_____

_____

Pray

Dear Jesus, I come to you right now needing to remember that you never leave me alone. Today, help me see that you are for me and with me in my journey. Psalm 118 tells me that you answer me in my distress, and sometimes your remedy for my surroundings is that you put me in a spacious place. So may I see that this space is from you to fill my heart with peace. The Lord is for me; I will not be afraid. What can man do to me? (Psalm 118:6). Because you are my helper, I will overcome through you (Hebrews 13:6). So help me, Lord, find my refuge in you today, for you are my strength and my song, my salvation and victory (Exodus 15:2).

Act

Reach out to a friend to share your feelings of loneliness. If you don't have someone like this, share with your husband and connect with our community through the website, join one of our support groups, or reach out on social media. It's important for you to have companionship on your journey, so choose a step to take today.

9

Inside the Pit

I sink in the miry depths, where there is no foothold. I have come into the deep waters; the floods engulf me.

Psalm 69:2

The sun sank below the dusty window ledge. I (Jenn) didn't bother getting up off the couch to turn on the lights. All I wanted was to stay curled up in my husband's arms, our toy poodle nestled against my neck. For hours, our little family sat there, grieving in the dark.

Going through a failed round of IVF crushed me. After months of trying other fertility treatments, my husband and I reluctantly decided to do IVF as a last-ditch effort at pregnancy.

Knowing the procedure had a 50/50 chance of success, I wasn't planning to rush out and buy a ton of baby clothes. I had prepared for the test to come back negative. I had *not* prepared to get a call from the doctor saying, "We didn't get any embryos."

No embryos. No baby. No hope.

This is where we hit rock bottom. Nothing had worked, and we were out of options. Without a clear path forward, my husband and I had to face reality: our dream of getting pregnant might never come true. I think of this place as the pit. You're overwhelmed, defeated by impossibility, wondering if God has abandoned you.

I'm sorry if you're stuck in the pit. I've been there too. Though I had been a Christian for a long time, infertility led me to doubt God. He had the power to give me a baby but chose not to. Exasperated, I asked him, "Why are you doing this, Lord? Have you forgotten me? Do you even care?"

At one of the worst moments of my life, I couldn't see God's goodness. In despair, I cried with the psalmist, "*You* have put me in the lowest pit, in the darkest depths" (Psalm 88:6, emphasis added).

Down and Doubting

As we've mentioned before, infertility is traumatic. Studies show that the psychological distress of infertility is similar to what cancer patients face.[1] In addition, both women and men going through fertility treatments are at greater risk for clinical depression.[2] These are real mental health struggles that require attention before they get too severe.

If you're experiencing chronic sadness affecting your day-to-day activities, please call someone and get help. God can provide healing through counselors, therapists, and medicine. Talk to a trusted friend who can give you support. When we're in the pit, we often need someone on the outside to throw us a lifeline.

Whether or not you're clinically depressed, you probably still wrestle with doubts. That's normal. We don't know the future because we're not God. So we ask questions and try to make sense of why he's allowing us to suffer.

The good news is that God doesn't scold us for questioning him. In the Old Testament, the psalmists, Job, and several prophets ask God "Why?" more than fifty times. You'd think the Creator of the universe would get annoyed after all that nagging. But God listened patiently as his people cried out for understanding in the midst of their turmoil.

Instead of revealing his reasons, God offered something better: truth about himself. Look at what he promises to be and do for his beloved children:

- He is in control. (Isaiah 14:24)
- He loves you with an everlasting love. (Jeremiah 31:3)
- He is your keeper. (Psalm 121:5)
- He created you for a purpose and has a future for you. (Jeremiah 29:11)

For every "Why?" you beg to know the answer to, God answers, "Look at me." As you grasp for explanations that might not come, turn to his Word and be reassured that you can trust him.

Talk to Your Feelings

Reading and meditating on Scripture can offer comfort when infertility stirs doubts. But even then, there are times when the darkness refuses to lift. We call out to God, but he seems distant, unmoved by our pain.

You don't need to be ashamed if you're feeling despair. Lord knows I've been in the pit more than once. And I can tell you what I've learned about speaking truth to our feelings.

God created us to experience emotions as part of his good design. Feelings help us communicate, relate to him and others, and express our worship. We don't need to hate our negative feelings, but we don't always need to believe them either. Like the rest of this world, our emotions are flawed. Physical problems, stress, genetic traits, or a combination of these and other issues can throw our feelings out of sync with reality.

As an example, think of a time when you were sick and had the chills. Even if the weather was warm and your thermostat was set to seventy degrees, you might have buried yourself under a pile of blankets. Your feelings were telling you something: "My body feels cold." But that message didn't match the actual temperature of your surroundings.

The truth is, no matter what we feel, God is always with us. Since time began, he's been moving toward his people—saving and forgiving, guiding and growing, restoring and transforming. Even after his people rebelled and turned their backs on him, God kept his promise: "I will never leave you nor forsake you" (Hebrews 13:5 NKJV).

Although your fertility struggles might make it seem that God is far away, he hasn't walked out on you. He sent Jesus to draw you close to him, to walk in the light where he lives.

Romans 8:38–39 guarantees that "neither death nor life, neither angels nor demons, neither the present nor the future, nor any powers, neither height nor depth, nor anything else in all creation, will be able to separate us from the love of God that is in Christ Jesus our Lord." "Anything else" includes everything that's hard about your journey.

In longing and heartbreak, in devastating test results and failed fertility treatments, in miscarriage and ectopic pregnancy and recurrent loss—through the worst of your waiting, God is *with* you and *for* you.

How Deep Love Goes

God stayed with me in my post-IVF depression. And he'll stay with you in your dark season, however long it lasts.

When doubt and despair press on your soul, remember that Jesus went to utmost lengths to save you. He is the greatest answer to our "whys," as pastor Timothy Keller pointed out in *Walking with God through Pain and Suffering*:

> Yes, we do not know the reason God allows evil and suffering to continue, or why it is so random, but now at least we know what the reason is not. It cannot be that he does not love us. It cannot be that he does not care. He is so committed to our ultimate happiness that he was willing to plunge into the greatest depths of suffering himself. He understands us, he has been there, and he assures us that he has a plan to eventually wipe away every tear. Someone might say, "But that's only half an answer to the question 'Why?'" Yes, but it is the half we need.[3]

Christ lived, died, and rose again to deliver you from the ultimate pit—separation from God. You've been rescued from sin and promised a sorrow-free home for eternity. So take comfort. The hopelessness of infertility can't defeat the certainty of the cross.

Reflect

• What has caused you to feel like you're in the pit? What seems to be keeping you there?

- What questions would you like to ask God right now?

_____

_____

_____

_____

_____

- What do you think about the idea of speaking truth to your feelings? Does it sound doable or impossible? Which specific truths would you tell your feelings?

_____

_____

_____

_____

_____

Pray

Dear God, this endless waiting for a child has dragged me to the lowest of lows. I'm sad and discouraged; it feels like you left me in misery. Thank you for letting me ask you questions. I need you to shine the hope of Christ into my despair. Give me faith that seeks to worship you more than wanting to know why you're allowing pain in my life. Lord, I believe; help my unbelief (Mark 9:24).

Act

Place a candle (real or battery-powered) next to your bathroom sink. Light it every morning while you get ready as a reminder that you always have hope because Jesus is always with you.

10

How Long, Lord?

How long, Lord? Will you forget me forever? How
long will you hide your face from me?

Psalm 13:1

Anger is a messy feeling. It can become overwhelming and downright ugly in a split second. Infertility made me (Kelley) angry because of all the unknowns. As the heartache dragged on, I fixated on one question: *How long must I wait for a child?* I battled this thought to keep it from becoming a fear. But it was hard not to feel exasperated when I just wanted the agony to end.

Sometimes anger begins with shock. Brooke explained how going through miscarriage shook her to her core, leading her to question God's very nature. "Suddenly, God felt unsafe, scary, and unpredictable. He was no longer trustworthy. Mentally, I ran from him, closing off my heart to the one I felt had inflicted such pain. I walked around for weeks telling everyone that God was simply mean. What else could I conclude after so many miscarriages?"

Our attempts to get pregnant and carry a baby show us how little we can control. Trying to conceive is just that—*trying.* No matter how much we try, conception is still in the sovereignty of God's will and creating hands. Therefore, it's easy for our waiting to make us angry at God, ourselves, our bodies, our husbands, or other people. We long for an explanation for our brokenness, and we seek a target for our intense feelings.

Jaclyn, my friend and our Waiting in Hope community director, shared honestly about where she directed her anger: "I was angry with God. Angry at his chosen silence. Angry that in my greatest pain, God felt so far off. I wondered what the point of having a personal relationship with God was if he was going to be silent. Why wasn't he making his comfort, his love, his goodness, and his peace tangible to me, his daughter, in my times of greatest need?"

The Source of Anger

Most of us feel guilty about being angry. We consider anger a destructive emotion that we shouldn't have or express. However, anger isn't necessarily a bad emotion. So let's start by investigating the source of our anger.

Anger can be holy and based on injustice. Throughout the Bible, prophets expressed anger and lament over the injustice done to God's people. Likewise, God stirs anger in us, often to prompt us to respond to an injustice or a need. Think about Jesus at the temple flipping tables because they were being used for unholy purposes (Matthew 21:12).

Infertility is a type of injustice. As we have seen, life is unfair due to the brokenness of this world. The sins of Adam and Eve brought all humans pain and hardship, including effects on our womanhood.

In Genesis 3:15–16, God said to the serpent (Satan), "'And I will put enmity between you and the woman, and between your seed and her Seed. . . .' To the woman He said: 'I will greatly multiply your sorrow and your conception; in pain you shall bring forth children'" (NKJV).

God knew Satan would hate women. However, it's essential to understand that one consequence of the fallen world is a tainted childbearing process. Intensified pain entered the story at the fall, but thankfully this wasn't God's original design or his end to this story or our story.

When our expectations are not met, it's okay (and normal) to be disappointed. It leaves us confused as our questions of disbelief grow each day. We can't possibly understand, make sense of, or control the instability around us. These unknowns can lead to festering anger. And through our questioning of these unknowns, our anger intensifies.

In my overwhelming anger, I wondered many times whether God saw me or cared, or, as Jaclyn questioned, was his silence his answer for my heart? Was he showing me I was alone even from him? As we learned in chapter 8, God has not left us, even when our emotions tell us otherwise.

The anger from our unmet expectations makes us believe we deserve different from what God is providing. Yet why do we think God owes us a life free of pain?

Isaiah 43:2 describes hardship as "when you pass through the waters," "when you pass through the rivers," and "when you walk through the fire." Notice that it's not *if* you will endure hardship, but *when*. The trials are stated as a given. Like Christ, we, too, will experience pain in this broken, sinful world. Jesus said in John 16:33 that we should expect pain and suffering in this world. Yet he is with us, overcoming the world and providing us peace.

The Direction of Anger

Years ago, Justin and I were experiencing frustrations and restless hearts regarding significant church situations, which led us to seek wise counsel. A trusted church pastor listened as we expressed our feelings, and he lovingly explained that God sometimes uses our frustrations and uneasiness to stir change in us.

He advised us to examine the cause of our feelings and warned us that anger could turn unholy if God is asking us to act and we do not. Wisdom is seeking God's leading to adjust, jump, or change courses before our feelings lead to outbursts of anger aimed at the church, God, or others.

Anger often seeks a target. It's an emotion that is directed toward someone or something. At some point, you've likely been angry at yourself, your body, your past, your future, your spouse, a friend, or a family member.

There is a safe direction for our anger, and that place is the Lord. Our Creator and King is good, strong, and faithful to handle everything, even anger. He allows us to express and vocalize our grief and frustration through the process of lament.

In *Dark Clouds, Deep Mercy,* pastor and author Mark Vroegop describes how learning to lament involves a kind of complaining that is biblical. "Through godly complaint we are able to express our disappointment and move toward resolution. We complain on the basis of our belief in who God is and what he can do."[1]

The books of Psalms and Lamentations give us examples for how to express lament. These prayers describe explosive feelings, even anger, that can lead us to God. Lament can become our pathway to God when life is hard or God feels far off. Most psalms of lament or sorrow start with anguish and build into confidence in God, resulting in praise toward him. "But God has surely listened and has heard my prayer. Praise be to God, who has not rejected my prayer or withheld his love from me!" (Psalm 66:19–20).

We can practice lament by following this same pattern.

- *Turn to God in prayer.* Bring your complaints and circumstances to him. Acknowledging that he is in control gives words to the tension between what we know about God and how we feel about him.
- *Ask God to act.* Ask God boldly to act on your behalf, believing that he is God and has good purposes for your pain and needs.

- *Choose to trust God.* This is an active surrender of your life to God and the beginning of acceptance as you release control over your unknowns. When you surrender to God, your questions find a place to go. Author Elisabeth Elliot described how she came to this place of acceptance: "Whatever is in the cup that God is offering to me, whether it be pain and sorrow and suffering and grief along with the many more joys, I'm willing to take it because I trust him. Because I know that what God wants for me is the very best."[2]

Your anger could be the catalyst God uses to draw you closer to him.

Lament Leads to Trust

In his laments of sorrow, David cried out, "How long, LORD?" (Psalm 13:1). Lamenting gives us permission to feel sorrow, acknowledge the real emotions, and rant to the Lord. Yet it doesn't stop there. Our protests are transformed into petitions and then praise.

These authentic and intimate prayers in pain lead to trust, a way to praise God through uncertainty and sorrow. The truth of who God is can reign when we honestly surrender and no longer pretend that everything is okay.

We can't know how long, but God does.

He hasn't forgotten you. How could he? You are his child, and that would be impossible for the God who sees and knows every last detail about you—from the number of hairs on your head to the dozens of pregnancy tests that made you burst into tears.

Though his face seems hidden, God has never left your side. Believe that the one who saved you will someday, somehow make this right too.

Reflect

- Have you ever shared laments of sorrow like David: "How long, LORD?" Explain.

_____

_____

_____

_____

_____

- Describe how you've been angry during your journey. Consider whether your anger has been directed at someone or something; then write about it.

_____

_____

_____

_____

_____

- What do you think about the concept of directing your anger toward God? How can lamenting to God be helpful in your pain?

_____

_____

_____

_____

_____

Pray

Pray this prayer of lament from Psalm 42:3–8 (ESV): Lord God, "my tears have been my food day and night, while they say to me all the day long, 'Where is your God?' These things I remember, as I pour out my soul: . . . Why are you cast down, O my soul, and why are you in turmoil within me? Hope in God; for I shall again praise him, my salvation and my God. My soul is cast down within me; therefore I remember you. . . . Deep calls to deep at the roar of your waterfalls; all your breakers and your waves have gone over me. By day the LORD commands his steadfast love, and at night his song is with me, a prayer to the God of my life."

Act

Start lamenting to God in your sadness, anger, and overflowing feelings. Yell out to him in your car, on a run, or in the shower. Sometimes it's helpful to hear your audible voice crying out to him as David did in the psalms. Then ask God, "Speak to me; I need to hear from you. What do you say about my pain?" Be silent and listen for his still, small voice (1 Kings 19:12) to whisper to your heart. If this is new for you, start reading the psalms for examples.

CLINGING
· TO ·
HOPE

✦

The Spiritual Journey

11

Not a Punishment

Therefore, there is now no condemnation
for those who are in Christ Jesus.

Romans 8:1

I don't deserve children. The thought struck Francesca as the doctor told her the lab results. For two weeks, she had treasured the knowledge of life growing within her. She and her husband had been overjoyed to finally see a positive pregnancy test after doing IVF. They were still processing the glorious news when Francesca started bleeding. Hospital tests confirmed that her HCG had dropped to zero. In an instant, the couple's excitement came crashing down.

Going through miscarriage led Francesca to question God. She wondered if he was angry with her for walking away from the faith when she was a teenager. After both her parents and grandma died, she had turned to alcohol and sex to numb the grief. Since then, Francesca had recommitted her life to Jesus. But she couldn't shake the feeling that infertility and miscarriage might be God's way of punishing her for her party years.

"Sometimes I feel that I messed up so badly, God is telling me, 'There's no chance I can give you kids, Fran, because you're a disaster.'"

A Common Struggle

Francesca isn't the only one who struggles with feeling as though infertility is God's punishment. When I (Jenn) asked this question in the Waiting in Hope Facebook group, several women admitted they have thoughts that God is punishing them even though they know it's not true. Similar to Francesca, some women assumed they were paying for past mistakes. Others thought that God was teaching them a lesson, their faith was too weak, or they hadn't done enough to "earn" a baby. All these thoughts begin with a common belief: *God is causing me pain because I sinned.*

Friend, I'm sorry if you're grappling with this belief. Infertility is hard enough without feeling as though God is unleashing his wrath on you. Before we go further, let's grab hold of truth. Jesus himself declared that whoever believes in him is not condemned (John 3:18). Paul echoed his Savior's words, "Therefore, there is now no condemnation for those who are in Christ Jesus" (Romans 8:1). No condemnation means no sentence of punishment. The wages of our sins have already been paid. Because of Jesus, all who put their faith in him stand innocent before God.

Because of Jesus, infertility is *not* a punishment.

God's Word has the power to release us from feelings of condemnation. By looking at what the Bible says about sin and pain, we can see three truths to help us bravely challenge the punishment lie.

Pain Doesn't Always Mean Punishment

Remember what we talked about in chapter 5 when Adam and Eve ate the forbidden fruit? Their sin broke God's good creation, bringing death to the newborn world. Because of the fall, the world is contaminated by sin and life doesn't fit according to our view of fairness. "Good" people go through awful experiences. "Bad" people get rewards they didn't earn. Pain affects everyone, even the faithful.

The Bible includes several examples of godly people who suffered. Job was blameless before the Lord, yet he lost his children and wealth and became so sick he wanted to die (Job 1–3:1). Elizabeth was righteous in God's eyes, but she couldn't get pregnant until way past her childbearing years (Luke 1:5–7). Then there was the blind man Jesus healed with a mud wash. The disciples asked who had sinned to cause the man's blindness. Jesus set them straight: "'Neither this man nor his parents sinned,' said Jesus, 'but this happened so that the works of God might be displayed in him'" (John 9:3).

Allow these stories to lift your spirits. Though you and I sin, we don't need to interpret pain as a slap on the wrist for some wicked thing we did. Instead, for reasons beyond our understanding, God is allowing us to feel sin's burden on the world—but only temporarily. He sifts circumstances through his hands, stopping some difficulties and allowing others to fall on us for our ultimate good. You can find relief knowing that the Lord is working through your infertility not to punish you, but to put his glory on display.

Jesus Took the Punishment for Us

If you're familiar with the Bible, you know that everyone sins and comes nowhere near God's glory (Romans 3:23). So although we shouldn't think of infertility as punishment, all of us do deserve God's judgment.

This is what makes grace amazing. Out of his deep love for us, God sent Jesus to be our perfect substitute. No one else could take our place except the sinless Son of God. Christ satisfied God's justice and erased our sins for good by giving his own life as payment.

Isaiah 53:5 offers a gritty explanation of what Jesus went through to save us. "But he was pierced for our transgressions, he was crushed for our iniquities; the punishment that brought us peace was on him, and by his wounds we are healed." Christ's sacrifice should affect the way we think about our childbearing struggles. Infertility and other difficult experiences can't be forms of punishment because Jesus took the punishment for us. He willingly endured unimaginable agony so we could have peace with God.

Let that good news wash over you like a cleansing shower. You have a Savior who took your sin and stood condemned for you. As feelings of punishment unsettle your soul, remember that when God looks at you, he sees only the perfection of his Son.

God Disciplines, Not Punishes, His Children

Jesus took our guilt and gave us his innocence before God. Though we're saved for eternity when we put our faith in Jesus Christ, sin still causes us to trip. We know the good we should do and sometimes want to do it. But we also have times when the other option seems so appealing, we cave in and do what we shouldn't.

To improve our resistance to temptation, we need training. Think back to when you were learning how to ride a bike. You probably had a parent or other adult teach you what to do and encourage you to keep practicing. As we mature in our faith, our heavenly Father teaches us how to both want and do what's good. This training involves discipline—an action intended to correct, shape, and guide.

I know that hearing about discipline can stir all kinds of emotions. But try to stay with me while I explain that God's discipline is *not* punishment. The difference between punishment and discipline comes down to the purpose of pain. Where punishment causes pain to enforce justice, discipline allows pain to foster growth.

The Message version of Hebrews 12:6 says, "My dear child, don't shrug off God's discipline, but don't be crushed by it either. It's the child he loves that he disciplines; the child he embraces, he also corrects." Notice how this verse describes the person being disciplined: *child*, *loves*, *embraces*. God loves his daughters and wants us to grow as women of character. He knows the best ways to train our spiritual muscles—ways that might even challenge and hurt us for a period of time.

Believe it or not, knowing about God's discipline can strengthen your hope. The heartache of infertility isn't your cross to bear. Jesus, your Redeemer, already paid for your sins. And now God your Father is training you in holiness. He's walking with you every painful step of the way.

Embrace Freedom

I hope this chapter gave you a huge sigh of relief. Any thoughts about God punishing you with infertility do not come from him. Through his Spirit, you can reject these lies and live in the freedom Jesus secured for you. Rather than wait in fear of condemnation, you can wait with confidence knowing God has forgiven and accepted you as his own.

Reflect

- How are you viewing God? Do you see him as a heavenly judge pounding his gavel on the clouds? A mean dad who's sending you to your room? Journal your thoughts and feelings toward him.

_____

_____

_____

_____

_____

- Can you accept that Jesus' sacrifice on the cross covered your sins completely? Or do you think you've made mistakes that are unforgivable or require further punishment?

_____

_____

_____

_____

- How do you view God's discipline? Is it different from what you consider to be his punishment?

_____

_____

_____

_____

Pray

Dear Father, going through infertility is hell. Worse than the pain itself is the feeling that you sent me here. I've made awful choices in my life, and now I'm afraid that's why I can't get pregnant or am having miscarriages or stillbirths. Give me faith to believe that you're not punishing me. Replace my thoughts of condemnation with reminders of Jesus' sacrifice that made me pure. Open my broken heart to accept your grace.

Act

Instead of listening to Satan's lies, fight to hear what's true about yourself. Instead of shaming yourself for past failures or choices, ask God to help you see yourself how he sees you (for example, *loved, beautiful, known, safe, treasured*, etc.). Then write that word on your hand with a permanent marker.

12

Praise Him Anyway

Because your steadfast love is better
than life, my lips will praise you.

Psalm 63:3 ESV

My poor husband didn't know what hit him. It was the second Christmas
in our infertility journey. Before visiting family and being bombarded with
questions, we decided to exchange gifts, just the two of us (Jenn and Colin).
As we sat by our sad-looking fake tree, he handed me a small box and smiled,
eager to see my reaction. No sooner did the wrapping paper touch the floor
than the explosion went off.

"This isn't what I want!" I screamed. In a rage, I hurled the jewelry case
across the room and stomped out the door. (Let the record show I was taking
Clomid at the time. So yeah, my mood wasn't exactly stable.)

At that moment, I was laser-focused on my desire for a baby. Colin had
picked out a necklace to help me feel beautiful, and I responded by blowing
up at him. Instead of appreciating his thoughtfulness, I resented him for not
being able to give me the gift I wanted more than anything: a baby.

This is similar to how we often approach God during our wait. We know
every good and perfect gift comes from our Father (James 1:17), and we can

bring our petitions to him (Philippians 4:6). Whenever we pray, our minds often drift to our heart's loudest cry: *Please God, just give me a baby!*

Be reassured. It's good for us to ask the Creator to create life. But if the main reason we seek God is to get something from him, we treat him as a means to an end. You and I need to appreciate God for who he is, not just what he gives. The Bible proclaims the excellence of the Lord in and of himself, apart from his works. "Great is the LORD and most worthy of praise; his greatness no one can fathom" (Psalm 145:3). As we behold God's character, we see the beauty of worshiping him, even in our pain.

Let's look at three reasons to move from only asking to always praising our great God.

He Deserves Our Praise

The Lord of heaven and earth is far more than a baby supplier. Verse after verse in Scripture says no one is like him. Just try wrapping your head around some of his divine traits: holy, righteous, almighty, all-knowing, eternal, ever-present.

Who else could declare I AM WHO I AM (Exodus 3:14)? Only Yahweh, "the LORD," whose name means "to be." He exists by his own power, and everything's existence depends on him.

While God doesn't need anything from us, he tells us to praise him. The book of Psalms includes more than 170 references to praising God and giving thanks to our King. "Come, let us bow down in worship, let us kneel before the LORD our Maker" (Psalm 95:6). On our knees, we tell God how awesome he is. Not the "I just won a $500 shopping spree" kind of awesome. The "stand at the edge of the Grand Canyon and feel how small you are compared to the immensity before you" kind of awesome.

God is so much higher than we can comprehend. He deserves our worship all day, every day. Though it can be a challenge to praise him when we're hurting, his worthiness doesn't depend on how we feel. I AM will always be I AM. So let his unchangeable nature be the anchor of your praise.

He Wants a Relationship with Us

Why do you love your husband? Because he buys you flowers or mows the lawn? These are reasons to be thankful for your spouse, but they're not the foundation of your marriage. You love him because he's him.

The same should be true of our love for God. Jesus said the greatest commandment is to love God with all our heart, soul, mind, and strength (Mark 12:30). God wants all of us, and he wants us all-in in our relationship with him. If we base our affections on what he can give us, that means our love is conditional.

Our Father already proved his unconditional love when he sent Jesus to take our place on the cross. Of course, we can't repay his grace or love him perfectly. We're human and he's God. He knows our weaknesses and forgives us through the cleansing blood of his Son. Still, God calls himself a "jealous God" (Exodus 34:14). As he did with the Israelites, he desires to protect us from pursuing other gods—meaning anyone or anything we prize more than him. In this holy jealousy, God claims us as his own.

As you grieve over the gift you long for, take a minute to breathe in these truths: The Lord of the universe wants a relationship with you. He delights in you and rejoices over you with singing (Zephaniah 3:17). Like any good father, he wants what's best for you. And nothing could be better than keeping close to him.

Give your devotion to the lover of your soul. Not because he has the power to give you a child but because you adore him.

Praise Is for Our Good

Our Creator made us to make much of him. Ephesians 1 says God chose, adopted, and redeemed us "for the praise of his glory" (v. 12). That means worshiping him is our life's purpose, privilege, and duty.

The word *duty* usually makes us think of a boring chore like washing dishes or paying bills. But when you read the Bible verses that talk about worship, it sounds far from boring. The psalms burst with vivid descriptions of praising God with singing and dancing, shouting and clapping, feasting and blasting a variety of instruments. In other words, we throw him a huge, noisy party.

God is kind to give us an assignment that's really a celebration. He commands us to praise him for his sake and ours. As John Piper said, "We get the mercy, God gets the glory. We get the joy, God gets the praise. We get the hope, God gets the honor. Such a deal!"[1]

How does getting joy sound to you right now? As we trudge through the valley of infertility, it can seem like there's nothing good happening in our lives. Worship helps us lift our eyes from the difficulties surrounding us and look to God for pure, lasting satisfaction. Even if you don't get the test results you want or hear good news from the adoption agency, you have someone to celebrate.

Come as You Are

Maybe you feel too sad to raise a hallelujah. That's okay. Praise him anyway. He knows what you're going through. Your emotions aren't a surprise to him nor too much for him to handle. He wants you to come *just as you are*—whether happy or mournful, energized or dog-tired, high with hope or collapsed in defeat.

Read Psalm 42:5 and gain confidence to worship the Lord, no matter your emotional state: "Why, my soul, are you downcast? Why so disturbed within me? Put your hope in God, for I will yet praise him, my Savior and my God."

Your Savior is the gift you need most. Let all that is within you praise his holy name.

Reflect

• What do you focus on when you pray? Be honest. Though God already knows, it can help to take a step back and look at what's capturing your attention.

_____

_____

_____

_____

_____

• In his book *The Knowledge of the Holy*, A. W. Tozer wrote, "What comes into our minds when we think about God is the most important thing about us."[2] What's your first thought when you think about God? Don't worry if you haven't given him much thought before your fertility struggles. He welcomes your seeking now.

_____

_____

_____

_____

_____

- How hard or easy is it for you to worship the Lord as you wrestle with grief? By worship, I mean giving God honor in what you do and where you find ultimate joy.

_____

_____

_____

_____

_____

Pray

My King and my God, all my longings are before you. I've asked you the same request so many times. Thank you for allowing me to draw near your throne. I confess to having a one-track mind and not giving you the praise you deserve. Please deepen my awareness of how wonderful you are, Lord. Increase my passion for worshiping you. As much as I yearn for the gift of a child, I want to love you most.

Act

Search for the "Waiting in HOPE - Songs of Hope" playlist on Spotify or create your own playlist of worship songs. Listen to the playlist when you're driving your car or doing chores. This will help you begin to shift your heart toward praising the Lord, even in the middle of your waiting season.

13

Waiting Is Worth It

The LORD is good to those whose hope is in him, to the one who seeks him; it is good to wait quietly for the salvation of the LORD.

Lamentations 3:25–26

You've likely seen the popular onesie proclaiming "Worth the Wait." Maybe you have one and are awaiting the cherished day when you can put your newborn in it to announce his or her birth.

It's beautiful to witness these celebratory shout-outs of what God has done. What an inspiration to see that someone's waiting and pain brought joy.

Perhaps you have this or another item like it that helps you get through every round of testing, treatment, or adoption interviews—a beacon of light in your waiting, reminding you to keep going. It's good for us to be hopeful and look forward to the day the waiting will be over—when you, too, can look into the eyes of your child, wrapped in your special item, and say, "I've been waiting for you."

While sweet, these moments tend to focus only on the outcome. Without realizing it, our hope is placed in the results. I (Kelley) believe there is more in your waiting season than the end. I've seen how waiting can have value beyond simply filling space between our current reality and desired outcome.

In the process of waiting, we can learn much about ourselves. If we allow it, these seasons can grow and purposefully change us. Our waiting can be worth it regardless of the outcome.

The Motivation of Desperation

The burden of waiting causes us to become desperate for relief. Our eyes turn upward and outward as we become aware of our inability to resolve or end our waiting. The following psalms remind us where we find our safe place:

- "God is our refuge and strength, an ever-present help in trouble." (Psalm 46:1)
- "I will say of the LORD, 'He is my refuge and my fortress, my God, in whom I trust.'" (Psalm 91:2)

The Bible is full of stories of God's people waiting. Over and over again, we see God use waiting to draw his people to himself. For instance, the Israelites wandered in the desert waiting for their promised land, and David fled from King Saul while he waited to be king. However, although the people in these examples were given God's direct promise of what was to come for them, we have no clear promise about future events in our lives. I often struggled with this and questioned God, "Why did they get to know, and I don't?"

But God reminded me that even though the Lord had told them what was to come, they still didn't easily trust, obey, and follow during their delays. As a result, they, too, became discontent in their waiting. Therefore, even if we knew why or when our waiting would end, it wouldn't necessarily make it any easier or smoother.

Let's also consider Jonah, who was swallowed by a big fish (we often say it was a whale), and three days later, God made the fish spit him out. Though Jonah's story is complex, I believe he wasn't in the belly of that fish just for a good Sunday school lesson. Instead, the dark three days Jonah was inside the pit of death refined and drew him back to God. In Jonah 2, we see Jonah's heart changed by understanding his need for God. He cried out to God in his waiting and returned to God's guidance.

Jonah had to be in the fish. God placed him there out of mercy. It was in the darkness of the fish that Jonah became desperate.

Waiting awakens us to recognize our need for God. It's here when we find ourselves out of control, outside our abilities, or attempting to change the situation. Then, like Jonah, we desperately need God to intervene and rescue us.

Even more than a divine intervention miracle or an answer to our pleas, we find in our waiting that our hearts are pulled toward Jesus. In turn, we become less focused on what God can do for us. We long for his power to show up, to be near and hold us tightly through the waiting. We see that in these moments of our lives, the Lord God is all we have.

Our seasons of delayed waiting stretch us to our breaking point, where we have no one else and can't carry on. We collapse at the Lord's feet, desperate for him to relieve our sorrows and sustain us in our ongoing disappointments. As humans, we are frail and need someone to cling to as the painful days go by. We realize we aren't able to fix or change our situation. Yet God is sovereign and can.

Jonah was swallowed up in God's provision and grace; otherwise, the storm and sea he was thrown into would have taken his life. Even though Jonah's circumstances didn't necessarily make sense to him, God was protecting him. No one could rescue Jonah except God.

God Knows Better

At the start of the new year, I typically take some time and ask the Lord for a word or theme to focus on. So it was only fitting that the year the Lord gave me the word *trust* would become the most challenging year of our infertility journey. It's clear that the Lord knew I needed to work on trusting him fully, and infertility would be the "whale" to get me there.

During that year, I was compelled to trust God as I never had before. Leaning on him became essential to my daily life. One Sunday in particular was the pivotal moment I finally dropped the facade that I was okay and had it under control on my own. I was at a significant roadblock that had life-changing implications. My fertility clinic halted all treatments until I received clear breast biopsies.

My new reality was hard to acknowledge. All I wanted was a baby, yet I was now facing the possibility of breast cancer. However, as Justin and I prayed that afternoon, God, in his steadfast loving-kindness, brought us to the same verses. Psalm 33:20–22 had become our source of strength and truth to stand on: "We wait in hope for the LORD; he is our help and our shield. In him our hearts rejoice, for we trust in his holy name. May your unfailing love be with us, LORD, even as we put our hope in you."

God had gently covered us in his nearness and prepared us for this day and situation. Then the Lord pressed on my heart, *Do you trust me, Kelley?* In my deep, deep agony, God used his Word and Spirit to confirm to my heart that I must "wait in hope" for him. He is my help and shield that I can *trust*.

I had taken over control and was pushing ahead on our journey without thought to God's will or direction for my life. I was not trusting. I was lacking ability to wait in him. But in God's sovereignty, he knew better. He knew what was to come and that if I didn't learn this now, then my secondary infertility and coming losses would be impossible to endure. I had been pushing ahead one month to the next, only giving God an obligatory check-in for approval on my next step.

Instead of waiting in hope for the Lord, I had made it clear that he was neither my help, my shield, nor my hope. My hope was in the next attempt, the next month, or whatever I thought was best as long as God didn't yell a loud, *No!*

But the Lord wanted more for me. He was kind to provide an opportunity that forced me to yield to him, to get my attention and halt my efforts. I had gotten lost, and he wanted to turn my heart and refocus my eyes toward him.

Our waiting season is about much more than what we wait for. It's always about our hearts in our waiting. The time we spend waiting on something (like a baby) can cause us to go deeper in our relationship and intimacy with the Lord. Like any friendship, it requires time to know and grow closer. God continually pursues a relationship with us, moving us toward a deeper connection with him. When you know the Lord your God more, then you'll trust and depend on him more. In God's hands, our waiting can and will be worthwhile.

The Value of Waiting

The cute onesie we one day hope to see our little one wear is fun. God knows I have a crib full of cute little items for the baby we pray will join our family through adoption. I know God can do this, and I pray he does for you and me. But even so, our waiting can be necessary and good for each of us.

Throughout the Bible God used waiting seasons to soften the hearts of his people. He taught the Israelites to depend on him while they wandered the desert for forty years. He prepared David to be king during his years of hiding from Saul. And we saw what he did with Jonah, who had a change of heart after sitting three days in the belly of a giant fish. Just as God's people learned over and over again, we can believe that our Creator has a purpose in our waiting seasons. He is our rescuer, the only God who saves.

The real issue becomes what you choose to believe during this season. Is God using your waiting to make it worthwhile? Or is the baby at the end the only way this season will have any worth and value to you?

It is never too late to invest in your waiting season. Choose the better alternative: waiting in hope for the Lord. In your waiting, you can find true purpose. Sometimes it feels like a waste when you're going days, months, and years without a child, but the waiting can reward us with a greater dependence on the Lord.

Inside the whale moments of life, we become desperate for God, which draws us to him. May we not waste this waiting time.

Reflect

- How have you been waiting? What will make this waiting worthwhile for you?

_____

_____

_____

_____

_____

- In what ways would you like your waiting season to be different? How can you find purpose right now in your wait?

_____

_____

_____

_____

_____

- How has your waiting pushed you to greater dependence on God? If this hasn't happened yet, ask him to show you your desperate need for him.

_____

_____

_____

_____

_____

Pray

Lord, help me to wait well. I don't know how to do that at this point of my journey, but I know you desire my whole heart and my earnestness to see you more than the baby. Like David said in Psalm 40, may I choose to wait patiently for you, Lord. You hear my cries, you know my heart, and you are *constantly turning to me, lifting me up out of this pit or the one I choose to make for myself. Help me not get stuck in distractions, Lord, by placing my feet on your solid ground. Lord, draw me in to wait with and in you.*

Act

Your act today is to do nothing when you want to do something. (I know—doing nothing goes against everything we're used to!) For example, when you want to google a symptom but it's not necessary, don't. Instead, choose to pray and trust.

14

Ready for Battle

Therefore put on the full armor of God, so that when
the day of evil comes, you may be able to stand your
ground, and after you have done everything, to stand.

Ephesians 6:13

It was dark as I (Kelley) ran up and down the stairs of my childhood home. Snakes were chasing me. Their slithering bodies were a terrifying sight that I saw night after night. Yet this experience was more than simply a nightmare. It felt and looked real even when I was awake. Now I can see these hard moments as far more than they appeared.

It was spiritual warfare, and I was the target. As with any good movie, there was a battle of good and evil, light and dark. Years later, when going through infertility, I realized I was the woman being hunted, and the goal was to capture me in fear.

Ephesians 6:12 says, "For our struggle is not against flesh and blood, but against the rulers, against the authorities, against the powers of this dark world and against the spiritual forces of evil in the heavenly realms." Since the early days of creation, this has been the story line.

To understand, let's look back at God's wondrous creation, both visible and invisible. In Genesis 1:31, God examined his creation and declared, "It is good!" Then by Genesis 3, we see the serpent deceiving our girl, Eve. Somewhere between the first and third chapters deception enters the story.

The being we know today as Satan was originally created by God as a guardian cherub named Lucifer, who was exquisite in beauty, wisdom, and influence in his high-ranking position in the angelic host. What happened? God described this change in Ezekiel 28:17: "Your heart became proud on account of your beauty, and you corrupted your wisdom because of your splendor. So I threw you to the earth." Now known as Satan, which means adversary or false accuser, he is a fallen spiritual being with power and a clear mission to steal, kill, and destroy (John 10:10). And his mission includes trying to mislead us during our waiting journey.

Against Us

There is a reason that many women and couples who endure infertility, miscarriage, and the wait for a child report feeling bombarded by temptations that provoke fear and create conflict, especially within marriages. Since this season is intricately connected to the big picture of God's design, it's also in the crosshairs of our adversary.

In God's conclusion of creation with the woman, Eve represented his glorious beauty. As women, our bodies were designed to bring forth life—a reflection of how God brought forth life in the act of creation. Beyond our physical makeup, we tend to be relational, nurturing, and heart-focused beings. The core of who we are and who God created us to be reveals his heart, character, and nature; therefore, Satan is opposed to us because we display God to the world. Thus, after Satan's own fall, in his jealousy of the beauty he once had and woman now possessed, he went after Eve in Genesis 3:1.

In their book *Captivating*, John and Stasi Eldredge wrote, "No explanation for the assault upon Eve and her daughters is sufficient unless it opens our eyes to the Prince of Darkness and his special hatred of femininity."[1]

The Evil One will use whatever he must to deceive, destroy, and bring death. He wants nothing more than to use your infertility, your pregnancy loss, and your waiting to tear your life apart, lead your heart to doubt, and wreck your marriage. He tries to use our pain and insecurity against us in an attempt to convince us we are broken, forgotten, unloved, and unworthy.

Unfortunately, Satan knows our weakness, and he uses our blind spots to lie, accuse, and distract us into believing his narrative. During your loneliness of infertility or loss, have you noticed him whispering lies to you like he did to Eve?

I know you're tired, but I want you to hear this first and foremost: "You are from God and have overcome them, for he who is in you is greater than he who is in the world" (1 John 4:4 esv). This is a promise we must remember.

Fighting Back

As I began to reject the lies and accusations aimed at me daily, I found it to be life-giving. There is a stark difference between what Satan wants you to believe and what God says of you.

- Satan's voice is condemning, shameful, unkind, and vague.
  - Lies often use absolutes like "never" and "always." *You'll never be a mom. You'll always be alone.*
- God's voice is loving, true to Scripture, specific, and sounds almost too good to be true.
  - Absolutes apply only to God and his character. "I am the Lord, and there is no other" (Isaiah 45:5).

- God defines you as "fearfully and wonderfully made," lacking nothing (Psalm 139:14).

Think back to how Jesus defeated Satan in the wilderness when he was tempted. When he heard something that didn't line up with God's truth, he knew it was a lie and declared Scripture over it. In the same way, when you hear and identify a thought as a lie, your strategy should be to call it out by saying out loud, "No! In Jesus' name, I refuse that." "Yell a loud *no* to the Devil and watch him make himself scarce. Say a quiet *yes* to God and he'll be there in no time" (James 4:7 MSG).

The Enemy must flee in Jesus' name. Jesus is the power of God in flesh who defeated death, darkness, and the sin of the world to win us back to God. I love Mark 1:27, which says of Jesus, "He commands even the unclean spirits, and they obey him" (ESV). Even the spirits scheming against us fall to Christ's authority. They must obey.

This spiritual battle is happening whether you want to admit it, see it, or believe it. Every day, it's aimed at your heart, hoping to take you away from God. Yet the battle is already won. Satan has been and will be ultimately defeated. Revelation 20:10 declares that Christ will throw Satan into the lake of fire. Jesus wins.

Our Weapons and Power

If we are to engage in this crucial battle, we need to gather our spiritual defense weapons and prepare. We will need to learn how to fight back and be ready. Thankfully it's not on us; the Lord is the one "who goes with you to fight for you" (Deuteronomy 20:4).

In Ephesians 6:11 Paul described our part in this spiritual battle as choosing to "put on the full armor of God." (I love the Amplified version of verses 10–20 for its detailed picture of us using all the tools, weapons, and strength God provides.) This command to put on spiritual armor signifies our need and dependence on God to protect us.

God can and will equip us daily for the battle raging against us through his Word, community, prayer, and the Spirit.

- *The Word.* God gave us Scripture as our sword of the Spirit. It is our weapon of defense. Where truth is, deceit is not. Therefore, the Word of God helps us to distinguish the lies from his truth.
- *Community.* God uses true community with other believers in our lives to teach us as we watch others before and around us in the faith. Even Jesus didn't live alone. He gave us an example by forming deep relationships with different people during his ministry on earth.
- *Prayer.* Talking to God is essential in building an intimate relationship with the Father. As we speak to him, engage with him, and live in constant communication with him, we become intimate with him. We do this by calling on the Lord during every moment and detail of our days. By living a life of prayer we choose to see him guide us, strengthen us, and steady us.
- *Holy Spirit.* Our Helper is God's power living in us as believers. God gives us the gift of the Holy Spirit to be our constant help, guide, and counselor. As with any good relationship the Spirit doesn't push in, yet he longs for an invitation to lead our adventure. This can be done by continually asking the Spirit questions to see what is happening in a situation. "Lord, what is at play in this emotion or hardship?" Then trust the Holy Spirit's leading.

These tools are available for us to access and gain protection continually as we are aware of the Enemy's patterns to defeat. Unlike God, Satan isn't an omniscient being and can't read our inner thoughts. However, he is a crafty student of humans. His warfare typically manipulates our wounds and insecurities to whisper lies and accusations at us, which we hear as confirmation of our pain. If we accept his twisted schemes as truth, then he gains a grip on our hearts.

Yet let's tread lightly because not everything is spiritual warfare, just as not everything is a miracle. (Jenn will talk about miracles in chapter 17.) We need to be cautious about calling instances of getting a sweet parking spot a "miracle." In the same way, a flat tire is not necessarily the work of evil forces. If we are extreme in these spiritual views, it's easy to be thrown for a loop by every negative thought and caught up in wrong beliefs (Ephesians 4:14). Instead, we should pray that God's truth and wisdom will be our steady guide.

God's Protection and Victory

Opportunities to grow in faith often go hand in hand with seasons of spiritual attack. I was afraid of this idea even as a little girl pretending my nightmare about snakes didn't happen. Yet this fear grew in the dark for years, continuing until the truth became undeniable.

I now can see how that little girl scared the Enemy more. You see, he fears what your heart through faith can do. What the Enemy intended for evil, God used for good (Genesis 50:20).

It's within these experiences that we get glimpses of God's mighty protection over us. Satan's clever attempts are limited by God's surpassing power and control. In Job's story, we see that God put Satan on a leash and only allowed him to go so far. Satan was *not* in control over Job's testing and hardship, even though they were his idea. It was God who allowed only so much to be sifted through his gracious hands to touch Job.

God's hand has always and will always protect you too.

Reflect

- Do you believe you are in a spiritual battle? Why or why not?

_____

_____

_____

_____

_____

- From what you learned in this chapter, is there anything the Lord is prompting you to try or change?

_____

_____

_____

_____

_____

- Is there someone you've been fighting instead of being on defense against spiritual attacks?

_____

_____

_____

_____

_____

Pray

Heavenly Father, I ask you to place a hedge of protection around me (and my spouse). Psalm 91 declares that you hide me from the Enemy in your shelter, for you are my refuge. Lord, you give me rest in your shadow, for you are my safe place. You will rescue me and protect me with your armor, not allowing the Enemy access to my mind, thoughts, heart, body, or surroundings. I know you answer my prayers when I ask because I love you and trust in you alone, my Lord. Thank you, God, for your divine protection.

Act

Read Ephesians 6:10–20 (in the Amplified translation, if possible). Then note or visualize what Paul described as our part in choosing to put on the full armor of God. He gives us protection; let's learn how to use it.

15

The New You

We all, with unveiled faces, are looking as in a mirror at the glory of the Lord and are being transformed into the same image from glory to glory; this is from the Lord who is the Spirit.

2 Corinthians 3:18 (CSB)

There are cramps, then there are cramps on steroids. That's what I called the spasms that tore through my abdomen every cycle my husband and I (Jenn) tried to conceive. Our fertility specialist diagnosed me with endometriosis two years into our journey. The disease not only made it tough for us to get pregnant; it also gave me digestive problems and cramps so bad I nearly threw up.

My doctor said I had two options: take ibuprofen on a schedule or go back on birth control. As you can guess, I opted to keep trying and dealt with the consequences. Month after month, I pushed through the hellish cramps, hugging my beanbag hot pack to survive.

Pain comes with being a woman. From ovarian cysts to fibroids and Pap smears to mammograms, we endure a huge range of uncomfortable experiences.

But you and I know that infertility takes pain to another level. Some of us live with the agony of endometriosis or PCOS. If you've lost a baby to miscarriage, it's possible you bled heavily for weeks. Most of the fertility tests and treatments we go through are painful, if not excruciating. No one enjoys bloodwork, pelvic exams, or getting injections in your belly or rear end.

I don't know how much pain you've suffered already. Between the physical and emotional distress, you probably feel pushed beyond your limits. To make matters worse, you might be surrounded by mom friends who gripe about pregnancy and postpartum effects. As they complain, you think, *I'd give anything for stretch marks.*

Good Work in Progress

During this painful journey, we yearn for transformation. We long to go from empty arms to full womb, from crushing silence to pulsing heartbeat, from childless to mama.

With our focus on the problems in front of us, we tend to pray that God will change our circumstances. These prayers are fine but shortsighted. We forget God's purposes go deeper than the results we hope to see. While we want God to change something *about* us, he wants to change something *in* us.

Philippians 1:6 says, "He who began a good work in you will carry it on to completion until the day of Christ Jesus." The "good work" the apostle Paul was talking about is God's continuing work of grace in the life of a Christian. God started this work when he rescued us from sin through Jesus' life, death, and resurrection.

As if saving us for eternity wasn't enough, God also gave us his Spirit, who helps us live in a way that pleases him. What pleases God is holiness. *Holiness* means being set apart by God, to God, for God's purposes. Without God, we can't live holy lives.

Are you noticing a pattern here? God is changing us to be holy like him. More specifically, he's conforming us to the image of his Son (Romans 8:29). Jesus is the exact imprint of God's nature, the radiance of his glory in a dark world (Hebrews 1:3). The more we become like Jesus, the more we grow into our new, glory-reflecting nature. As Paul wrote, "Therefore, if anyone is in Christ, the new creation has come: The old has gone, the new is here!" (2 Corinthians 5:17).

These verses can give you hope as you suffer the ache of infertility. God is working in you through your waiting. The days that pass with nothing but pain aren't a waste. Because he loves you, God wants to transform you. All the pulling, twisting, prodding, and stretching has a purpose to form you into a dazzling new creation.

Our Spiritual Makeover

At this point you might be wondering what you're changing into. What will this new woman look like? How will she talk, think, and act? Or perhaps you feel stuck in the pain, angry, frustrated, or unworthy of being transformed.

The Bible uses a relatable metaphor to explain how we're becoming like Jesus. In Colossians 3, Paul said that those who commit their lives to Jesus get a wardrobe makeover. If you've watched any fashion reality shows, you know how this starts. The designer checks out the person's closet, offers a scathing critique, then with a look of disgust dumps the person's old clothes in the trash.

In our spiritual makeover, we take off our old, sinful selves and put on our new, Christlike selves. The old self includes the ways we give in to temptation. While we're saved through faith in Jesus, we still struggle with saying no to wrongs such as greed, rage, lust, hatred, and foul language.

To get rid of our old selves, we have to "put to death" these lingering sins (Colossians 3:5). Other verses talk about dying to ourselves. Yes, this sounds drastic. But think about your worst bad habit. It would probably take extreme measures to quit something that ingrained in your muscle memory.

Dying to ourselves is painful. We want to be the boss of our lives and have everyone else follow our lead. Being remade in the image of Jesus means making him Lord—we love what he loves, and we hate what he hates. As we toss the dirty rags of our old self, we don't stay naked. We choose the hard no to embrace the better yes.

Saying yes to Jesus' ways allows us to put on the new self. "Therefore, as God's chosen people, holy and dearly loved, clothe yourselves with compassion, kindness, humility, gentleness and patience. Bear with each other and forgive one another if any of you has a grievance against someone. Forgive as the Lord forgave you. And over all these virtues put on love, which binds them all together in perfect unity" (Colossians 3:12–14).

This is who you're becoming: a beautiful soul. Through you, God will showcase his glory to those around you. Imagine how you can display these qualities while you wait:

- *Compassion* as you support others who are hurting.
- *Kindness* toward doctors, nurses, social workers, and other people you interact with.
- *Humility* as you serve your church and neighbors.
- *Gentleness* when you respond to baby shower invitations.
- *Patience* with your spouse during hard conversations.
- *Forgiveness* toward those who tell you, "Just relax."
- *Love* for Jesus, your living hope.

Time to Grow

Transformation is a process, and a process takes time. We of all people know that taking time hurts. Yet our pain has purpose. God uses time to grow us through a slow, continual renovation. "Therefore we do not lose heart. Though outwardly we are wasting away, yet inwardly we are being renewed day by day" (2 Corinthians 4:16). God wants to make you new. We don't simply wait in our infertility, but we choose to wait in hope. Our confidence is that he can use our waiting season to make us more like Christ.

Let this truth cheer your heart. Though infertility may be breaking you physically and emotionally, the Spirit of God is infusing resurrection into your spirit. He's giving you new desires, new habits, a whole new way to live life, the way you were meant to be.

Reflect

- How do you think about the pain of infertility? Are you a "no pain, no gain" person, or do you see pain as an obstacle that you need God to remove?

_____

_____

_____

_____

_____

- Have you thought much about the inner transformation God might be doing through your waiting? Why or why not?

_____

_____

_____

_____

_____

- What are some ways you can clothe yourself with Christlike qualities?

_____

_____

_____

_____

_____

Pray

Dear Lord, you know the pain I've been suffering. Between my physical and emotional health, I feel stretched past my limits. While I ache for you to change my circumstances, I know you're working on shaping me to be like Jesus. Give me patience as you complete the good work of transforming me from the inside out. Let your grace flow through my motives, thoughts, and actions, even as I press on in the wait.

Act

Read Colossians 3, and make a list of the traits of the new woman God is creating you to be. Use a dry-erase marker to write one quality on your bathroom mirror. When you see your reflection, you'll have an idea of who you are becoming.

16

My Story, His Story

He has saved us and called us to a holy life—not
because of anything we have done but because of
his own purpose and grace. This grace was given us
in Christ Jesus before the beginning of time.

2 Timothy 1:9

"I wouldn't wish this [infertility] on my worst enemy." I've heard this a million times. And it's accurate. I (Kelley) would never have chosen this journey for myself.

This is not the story you or I would have written or ever dreamed of for our lives, but here we are on a path chosen for us. I don't know why you are on this undesired life detour, but I believe there's more going on than what you can see.

Most women I meet through Waiting in Hope Ministries wrestle with the idea of infertility being their story. We all want our lives to follow a more straightforward, expected plan, like an A + B = C equation.

I wish it worked that way. It would be great if we had an easily determined road map without unknowns, fears, and any of the concerns that accompany our journeys to parenthood. Yet everyone's story and experience of infertility, miscarriage, and waiting for a child looks different. None of us will walk through this season with the same journey, and each of us has a unique path to take.

Infertility in the Bible

It's encouraging to hear the stories of other women who understand this infertility journey, especially when I witness inspiring success stories. I find it particularly encouraging that God included at least seven infertile women in Scripture.

God cared for barren women so much that several of them were chosen to be included in his grand story of salvation written for us to see. He continues to show his power and goodness in ways that are unique to each woman's story, including your own.

From Sarah to Hannah to Elizabeth, a similar narrative is written of redemption. Their stories, although complex and heartbreaking, especially in light of their culture's cruel treatment of barren women, were still purposefully woven into God's story for all his people.

Sarah

Abraham's wife, Sarah, spent most of her life without a child and finally gave birth to her promised son, Isaac, at ninety years old (Genesis 12–21). At first, she didn't believe God's promise to make Abraham a great nation—she even laughed in skepticism. But God did not waver in his plan, even when Sarah took matters into her own (sinful) hands to give Abraham offspring.

I imagine those thirteen years between the promise and fulfillment of a child must have been trying times in her waiting. But although Sarah was older, nothing proved impossible for God. Sarah made mistakes, yet God used those mistakes to help her to learn to trust in his timing.

God did not waste her waiting but gave it purpose. His plan was more extensive than her view. Sarah didn't know that her descendants would be so numerous that she would become the mother of the nation of Israel, as promised, through her son, Isaac.

Hannah

Hannah is most known for praying and then conceiving. Unfortunately, she's often misunderstood, and her story is misinterpreted to mean "If you pray and have faith like Hannah, then you'll get pregnant." But God is not a genie who must grant us our wishes. Instead, Hannah's story reveals a glimpse that God is more concerned with our hearts in our waiting.

We are told that Hannah was seen and remembered by God: "The LORD remembered her" (1 Samuel 1:19). We see her vulnerability and desperation bring her to her knees at the temple. Her focus shifted off her pain and onto her God.

Hannah became more focused on where her waiting was taking her heart. By 1 Samuel 1:15, we see her pouring out her soul before the Lord at the temple. During her prayer, Hannah wept so bitterly that the priest even thought she was drunk (I imagine that was some serious ugly crying). But in her prayer, she surrendered her story to join in God's story, vowing to trust God with her son (1 Samuel 1:11). The Lord answered Hannah's prayers, and she gave birth to Samuel, who would become the last of the judges of Israel and anoint King David of the royal line leading to Christ Jesus.

I love that we get to see our girl Hannah become dependent on God. Finally, in her pleading, she realized that he was writing her story and that she could trust him even with her deepest desire for a child.

Elizabeth

Elizabeth had to wait decades for her child. Luke 1:6–7 describes her as upright and blameless—yet barren. Was there purpose in her waiting? Scripture says, "Elizabeth was not able to conceive, and they were both very old" (v. 7). Then the remaining text in Luke 1 describes the encounter her husband, Zechariah, had with an angel of the Lord about his coming son. This son was to be John the Baptist (you may recognize his name). Of course, it was key that John the Baptist come at the exact right time to prepare the way for Jesus Christ to rescue the world.

We see God's purposes still being prepared for Elizabeth even during her many years without a child. It was in her waiting that God was working. It wasn't her fault; it was God's will. Elizabeth's "why?" had a greater God-glorifying purpose than mere waiting.

The Subject of Your Story

We see that God brought critical figures in his rescue plans from these women whose wombs could not conceive. He cared about their individual stories. He remembered them, worked through their pain, and gave them significant parts to play.

God saw these barren women, whom their society viewed as worthless and cursed. And to those who felt their story hadn't started, God flipped the narrative, proving their stories mattered greatly.

Somewhere in the middle of my story, I found a better story—God's story. I'd become worn out from my attempts, efforts, and a misguided mentality of "I must do this because so-and-so did it." Instead, I began asking God what he wanted for me, for our marriage, and for our future. I started not just taking my needs to him but expanding my prayer life to be about all things, not just infertility and a baby. As my prayers deepened, I began to see glimpses of God at work.

I realized I could allow God to use this journey and join him in his work toward others. This step helped me accept my story.

I've heard some claim, "All barren women of the Bible got what they asked for." However, we have to be careful not to take any biblical story or passage out of the full context of God's Word and intentions. The Bible doesn't promise us that God will give us everything we ask for.

The Bible is not an ancient story but *the story* of all life. God used unlikely and infertile women in the Bible to remind us that he can and will use our stories too. Our infertile sisters of the Bible remind us that God's greater story can always be trusted and is more vital than our plans could ever be.

Your pain and this journey are *not* actually about you. I know that sounds insensitive, but hear me out. The grand story has always been about Jesus and his redemption of God's people. He not only wants to rescue you from your infertility but ultimately to reclaim your heart. God chooses to use your life story—even the most challenging parts—for his purposes and glory to point to Jesus.

His Glory Inscribed Through Your Life

When you realize that your story is bigger than yourself and that God is bringing redemption through your infertility struggles, you will experience the joy of watching his glory unfold.

Let's consider the implication of only living from our story. For instance, what would have happened if our biblical barren sisters had only seen their small tale and had not turned their hearts and eyes to the Lord's plan for them? Would they have been a part of God's masterful rescue plan that stretches all the way to you and me through Jesus?

He is the same God for you now as he was for them. He can be trusted even when we cannot see the plan, pathway, or purpose. God said in Isaiah 43:7 to bring "everyone who is called by my name, whom I created for my glory, whom I formed and made" (ESV).

The story God is already writing with your life isn't just your story. It's his story in and through you for his glory and kingdom here on earth. It's more significant than what we can see, understand, or fathom, and it is ultimately for our good. Jenn and I never imagined we would be writing a book about our struggles at the time (we didn't even know each other until years later). But in God's tender workings we saw how he was allowing us to relate to and support others in their waiting.

I don't know about you, but I'm glad he thought to add these barren women and their journeys into his story to remind us of his greater, loving picture.

Reflect

- What has your story looked like so far? Do you see purpose from any of it?

_____

_____

_____

_____

_____

- In what ways have you seen your story being used for someone else?

_____

_____

_____

_____

_____

- Have you shared your story with others, publicly or privately? If so, explain how and why.

_____

_____

_____

_____

_____

Pray

Lord, I want to believe and see that you are using my story. This pain I'm experiencing is more significant than me and my view. Lord, show me glimpses of my story being written for you, for others, and ultimately for your glory on this earth. I desire for these aches to have an eternal purpose. Jesus, help me surrender my heart, as the barren women in the Bible did. I trust you have determined my time spent here and this exact place where I live to help others and myself seek you, God (Acts 17:26). I want to trust you in my waiting and to see that your purposes in my story are better than my desires or plans.

Act

If you haven't shared your story of trying to conceive, pray about how you could do that in the next few days.

Share with your community. Do this publicly on social media or privately with one or two people. The goal here is to share and use your story outside yourself. God will move through your step of obedience even as you continue to wait.

Then write down your feelings about sharing and what happens when you do.

17

What a Miracle Looks Like

By his wounds you have been healed.

1 Peter 2:24

If someone held a contest for the most misused word ever, I (Jenn) would vote for *miracle*. (Although *blessed* is a close second.) I've always thought of a miracle as a jaw-dropping work of divine intervention—something along the lines of parting the sea or turning water into wine. So when people say things like, "It's a miracle I passed the test," I tend to roll my eyes.

The worst example of this happened at a low point in my infertility journey. Our small group leader had asked us to share answers to prayer, and one guy shot up his hand and gushed, "I was running late to work this morning and prayed that God would help me get there on time. You won't believe it—I hit green lights the whole way! What a miracle!"

It took all the restraint I could muster to keep my mouth shut instead of screaming what I felt: *I'm here, begging God to enable me to get pregnant after three years of failed fertility treatments, and you're calling an easy commute a* miracle? *Really?*

You don't have to be a word snob to understand why I got upset. For those of us who struggle with infertility, *miracle* has a specific meaning.

It's our number-one prayer request, the wish we make as we blow out the candles on each passing birthday. And we know it will take God's matchless power to provide healing and to work a miracle inside us.

Dear one, I know how deeply you yearn for a miracle baby. Maybe someone has encouraged you to "claim your miracle." Or perhaps you come from a faith background that believes miracles don't happen anymore. With so many views on miracles, what should you expect? Your heart begs to know what a miracle looks like.

A Miracle Looks Like Physical Healing

When we're talking about miracles, it's important to recognize the physical side of infertility. The problem isn't all in your head or simply due to stress. According to health professionals, infertility is a disease caused by medical issues with you or your husband, or a combination of factors that prevent pregnancy.[1]

Because infertility is a physical issue, we're asking God for physical healing. Whatever the diagnosis—PCOS, abnormal sperm, or the dreaded "unexplained infertility"—we need God to restore our reproductive systems to work the way he designed.

We're right to believe that God is our healer. After God delivered the Israelites from slavery in Egypt, he called himself "the LORD, who heals you" (Exodus 15:26). And as he told Sarah in Genesis 18:14, nothing is too hard for him—even enabling pregnancy for a woman of extremely advanced maternal age.

The New Testament also gives examples of God curing sickness and physical problems. Of all the miracles Jesus performed during his ministry on earth, some of the most dramatic were the times he healed the sick. He made the blind see, the lame walk, the deaf hear, and the lepers clean with a mere word or touch.

The Bible makes it clear that Jesus performed miracles to confirm he was the Son of God. As Peter proclaimed in Acts 2:22, "Fellow Israelites, listen to this: Jesus of Nazareth was a man accredited by God to you by miracles, wonders and signs, which God did among you through him, as you yourselves know." Not only did Jesus do this to display his authority, but his heart motivated him to heal. He was moved by compassion more than once when he saw people desperate for relief from their pain and suffering (Matthew 14:14).

The question isn't whether God *can* heal us from infertility but if it's in his will for us. If so, we can't predict how or when his healing will come. He might choose to enable natural conception. Or he might work through medical fertility treatments or alternative therapies. His timeline could take months or years. However, he might choose a different path, and the physical healing will wait until heaven.

Not knowing God's timing is hard for us. We'd rather get answers instantly. Though we can't read God's mind, he invites us to ask for healing. James 5:14 says, "Is anyone among you sick? Let them call the elders of the church to pray over them and anoint them with oil in the name of the Lord."

I hope this reassures you that it's good to ask God to heal your infertility. While he doesn't promise physical healing in every circumstance, he wants us to honor him as the ultimate authority over our bodies. You can come before his throne, seeking life from the Author of life.

A Miracle Looks Like Spiritual Healing

Picture how Jesus responded to those who begged him for healing—welcoming their neediness, meeting their eyes with mercy. But as much as Jesus tended to physical problems during his ministry on earth, there's something he cared about more. Jesus suffered and died not just to rid us from colds and cancer. He wanted to heal us *forever*. His death and resurrection provided a cure from the deadliest disease—our sin-sickness.

We see Jesus' concern for our spiritual health in the story of the woman with a bleeding disorder. Jesus told her, "Daughter, your faith has healed you" (Luke 8:48). This verse can be literally translated as "your faith has *saved* you." Notice Jesus said this to the woman after she stepped out of the crowd, trembling, and admitted why she touched him. The woman believed in her heart and confessed with her mouth that Jesus was Lord (Romans 10:9). Through faith in him, she received forgiveness from her sins. While she reached out to Jesus hoping for a temporary physical cure, Jesus gave her spiritual peace with God that would last for eternity.

Even as you ache for God to work a miracle in your womb, don't miss this deeper layer of his healing. The miracle we need most is for Jesus to bring us from death to life. Sin poisons our hearts and separates us from God. Out of love for us, he sent Jesus to live a perfect life, die a horrible death, and overcome the grave—all so that we could have a right relationship with God.

While your wait for a baby might continue, you don't have to wait for the miracle of being reborn. If you know Jesus, you're alive *now*. His Spirit is in you, guiding, comforting, and empowering you to grab hold of resurrection hope.

His Deeper Answer

Author and speaker Joni Eareckson Tada knows what longing for a miracle feels like, though she can't feel anything from her shoulders down.

After a diving accident left her a quadriplegic at age seventeen, Joni became fixated on the story of Jesus healing a sick man by the pool of Bethesda. Every time someone read her the verses in John 5, a scene played out in her mind like a movie on a continuous loop. She was at the pool with other disabled people, waiting for Jesus to notice her, crying out, "Jesus, it's me . . . Joni! Don't forget me." But he didn't see her and passed by.

Joni gradually worked through her anger at God. Thirty years later, she and her husband traveled to Jerusalem and visited the ruins of Bethesda. There, Joni prayed and realized Jesus *had* seen her and answered her prayer:

> Lord, your no answer to physical healing meant yes to a deeper healing. And a better one. Your answer has bound me to other believers and taught me so much about myself. It's purged sin from my life, it's strengthened my commitment to you. Forced me to depend on your grace. Your wiser, deeper answer has stretched my hope, refined my faith, and helped me to know you better . . . I know I wouldn't know you . . . I wouldn't love and trust you . . . were it not for this wheelchair.[2]

You can experience this healing too. Commit your life to Jesus, whether for the first time or as a renewal of your faith. (If you haven't already made a commitment to Jesus, read "How to Put Your Faith in Jesus" at the end of this book.) Marvel at the depth of his love, how he died on a cross to save you. For by his wounds, you have been healed (1 Peter 2:24).

Reflect

- What comes to mind when you hear the word *miracle*? Be as specific as possible.

_____

_____

_____

_____

_____

- What do you think of the concept of God as your healer? Do you think that he owes you healing if you have enough faith, that he no longer heals supernaturally, or that he only cares about your soul and not your body? How has this chapter affected your perspective?

_____

_____

_____

_____

_____

- How often do you think about your need for spiritual healing? What work has God done in your heart?

_____

_____

_____

_____

_____

Pray

Lord, I know nothing is impossible for you. You're a wonder-working God, the creator and sustainer of life. My husband and I need your healing touch to restore our fertility and form a little human in my womb. Draw us toward your will, whether that means pregnancy, adoption, or another path. Wherever you lead, help me trust your timing. Give me a heart awed by your miracle of salvation. Romans 11:36 reminds me that all things are from you, through you, and for you, including my body and soul.

Act

List on a piece of paper how you've been expecting God to work a miracle through your infertility. Now I'm about to ask you to do something—please know I'm asking with tenderness: I want you to rip up that paper. It's time to surrender to God what you think your miracle will look like. Instead, come to God with open hands, and let him define the miracle he has for you.

18

Eyes on Eternity

But our citizenship is in heaven. And we eagerly
await a Savior from there, the Lord Jesus Christ.

Philippians 3:20

I (Kelley) wish I knew them. I long to hold them in my arms and smell their scent. I will never fully understand why they're not here. After two of my miscarriages, I tried hard to accept my reality. However, I had a lot of questions and began pondering the "whys" even though it was entirely beyond my comprehension. I pleaded to God for understanding as I ached and missed my babies. In a moment of clarity, the Lord impressed upon my heart these words: *I have them.*

I know this to be true, yet it struck me. The two miscarriages happened a year prior to when my now living son was conceived—oddly comforting timing. I heard echoing in my heart, *These are different babies*, almost as clear as an audible voice from the Lord. It was then that I realized that if those two babies were here as I had desperately pleaded to God for, then my son would not be. He is not them. Let me be clear: in no way does my living son replace the void or pain of my children gone too soon. Instead, this clarity seemed to bring light to a sad and dark spot, as I felt the Lord in his loving comfort whisper, *I'm holding them.*

I know these are impossible things to grasp, and you may be frustrated reading my personal story. I get it. I've been there. I simply want to share a picture of what God revealed to me. The Lord provided much-needed peace and comfort by helping me look to heaven, which I would need as I endured my third miscarriage with secondary infertility a few years later.

Not many things on earth can cause us to look forward to heaven like waiting for a baby and trying to grow a family. We long for the pain to end, to regain what was lost, and to see wrongs made right.

Made for Heaven

I used to think of heaven in simplistic images like a hazy fog of light and floating around on clouds. But as I've gotten older and grown in my faith, I've realized that heaven is far beyond my comprehension and expectations. God's grandeur cannot be limited to my imagination.

Your view of heaven might be grand or an obscure idea you contemplate only at funerals. But for believers, heaven holds much more for us than clouds. It's not just where we go when our days on earth are gone. Heaven is the place where the Lord God dwells.

If we believe in Jesus as our Lord and Savior, then heaven is everything to us. In his ultimate victory, Jesus conquered death (our death) and took our place, thus freeing us to spend eternity with him in heaven. "Because we know that the one who raised the Lord Jesus from the dead will also raise us with Jesus and present us with you to himself" (2 Corinthians 4:14).

It's in Christ that our passing from this earth actually leads to our greater life in heaven. If you've been in the church for even a short time, you've probably heard, "This is not our home." Earth, the way it is now after the fall, was not God's intent for us. Our true home is with God, our Creator and Father. Our hearts were created to be with God.

It's as though we have a deep sense at our core that the pain, loss, and aches on earth are not right. At funerals, we might hear, "She/he shouldn't be gone," and, "This isn't okay." These phrases echo a similar notion we profoundly sense: *This isn't how it's supposed to be.*

In the original creation described in Genesis, Adam and Eve walked in the garden with God (3:8). Can you imagine what it would have been like to experience God's nearness and presence in that way? God's design and intent have always been to be with us.

Our eternal nearness to God in his presence is what we were created for. "He has made everything beautiful in its time. He has also set eternity in the human heart; yet no one can fathom what God has done from beginning to end" (Ecclesiastes 3:11).

Our Pain Is Temporary

We know all too well that our longings for a baby can cause us to focus inward on our waiting, our struggle, and our pain. I quickly became the victim in my own life, trapped in this reality I didn't choose. My shortsighted view made me angry at the world, God, and everything else that led me here.

I was totally self-focused, and it became impossible to see the big picture, let alone anything God could be doing in the process. My pain and my need for things to be different were all I could see. My intense longing for a baby quickly turned my eyes away from anything more significant. It's hard to see the whole picture when we zero in on our missing pieces. Yet eternity has a way of turning our eyes toward God's purposes and our greater promise.

Eternity can hold your pain in this waiting room. In heaven God will right the wrongs of this world and restore our pain and losses. We hurt now, but redemption is coming. "And after you have suffered a little while, the God of all grace, who has called you to his eternal glory in Christ, will himself restore, confirm, strengthen, and establish you" (1 Peter 5:10 ESV).

Because of eternity, we realize that the pain we experience is not God's original design for us, and it will not be with us forever. Our pain will not last. Our waiting season is only for a moment in light of eternity.

Paul understood this. In 2 Corinthians 4:18, he reminded us, "So we fix our eyes not on what is seen, but on what is unseen, since what is seen is temporary, but what is unseen is eternal." Paul often viewed his pain in this world in light of God's loving-kindness and the eternity awaiting. He knew that his pain would not last and that life with Christ is better than anything we could ever imagine here.

Since God promises his children that there is eternal life waiting for us, we know our pain is not forever but temporary. Therefore, God's big story (including our aches), written in us and around us, will be made right in eternity.

God's plans for us have an everlasting, holy purpose we can't always see or know. Although this is a brutal reality to wrestle with during our waiting season, we can decide to trust that God, in his loving care, is making a masterpiece with us in mind, even though we are finite and can only see but a speck of it.

Hope in the Unseen

God promised in Revelation 21:4 that in heaven, he will wipe every tear from your eyes; there will be no more death, mourning, crying, or pain. He will make everything new forever in the new heaven and new earth. Eternity holds our everlasting healing.

Thinking about eternal life doesn't magically make our pain disappear, but it can give us comfort in our unknowns. We grieve and miss our loved ones here on earth. Yet, as we focus our eyes on the home Jesus is preparing for us, it can change how we look at our current waiting room.

Regardless of the pain we experience in this life, Jesus' outstretched arms will hold us for eternity, when we will be with our babies who were gone too soon and walk hand in hand with Jesus for eternity, forever healed and made perfect. Having our eyes on eternity gives us hope in the unseen.

Reflect

- What do you envision when you think about heaven?

_____

_____

_____

_____

_____

- Did this chapter give you a new picture of eternity? How so?

_____

_____

_____

_____

_____

- How would your heart be different if you began seeing heaven as your eternal home? Would it cause you to wait differently?

_____

_____

_____

_____

_____

Pray

Heavenly Father, I long to be with you in heaven, to see you and my babies, my loved ones, and my friends gone from this earth. Help me to perceive my waiting and aches in view of your heavenly plan and picture for my life. Give me eyes to see and a mind to fathom that you love me enough to send Jesus to die for me and provide an eternal home. Your love is grand, and your love for me is grander. So, Lord, fill my heart with longing to be with you in heaven and not just for my season to end.

Act

Think of a difficult infertility memory, then picture Jesus with you at that moment. Jesus is eternal and will continue to be with you for the rest of your wait.

If you have lost a baby (or babies), I encourage you to visualize them with Jesus. Ask God to give you a glimpse of what this might be like for your baby (or babies).

19

Counting It Joy

May the God of hope fill you with all joy and peace
as you trust in him, so that you may overflow
with hope by the power of the Holy Spirit.

Romans 15:13

After years of disappointment, I (Kelley) had learned not to touch the mail.
I knew better, and yet I grabbed the envelope from the stack of mail. There
it was, the photo of a cute newborn with the words, "Meet our little bundle
of joy!"

People often use that phrase to describe a baby, as though that is where
joy is. Yes, a baby can bring joy to your life. So many things can spark joy
within us—but they can't be the ultimate source of joy in our lives.

Have you ever met someone who exudes joy, peace, love, and life in all
they do? My beloved grandmother Martha was that kind of person. Her life
was filled with trials and heartaches, but she seemed to experience joy in all
situations. Martha's life was a TED Talk example of joy. Even as her mind
started to go, she remained steady and grateful to be alive, praising God.
Her joy didn't waver, and she was not easily rattled or stressed. Even in an
unhappy situation, her peace remained.

What was her secret? What made her life and heart so different from others'? Jesus was the joy of her life.

Oftentimes, we look for immediate gratification and rescue from our problems in this outcome-driven world. We fall into the trap of seeing life as a simple formula: *Do this; get that.* Unfortunately, that perspective doesn't lead to a fulfilling or joyful life.

Our days of waiting for a baby can become consumed by all things baby and all the attempts we make to get a baby. But these efforts don't necessarily bring forth joy or life for us.

Tracking and counting become our full-time job. We count fertility shots, medications, the time between intercourse, appointments, and home studies. These efforts make any feeling of happiness difficult, let alone the far-fetched concept of joy.

The truth is, the joy we need isn't attached to an outcome.

The Source of Joy

Our understanding of *joy* and *happiness* has become complicated. They're not the same, yet they are often used interchangeably (including in the Bible). Even now, my spell-check tries to do just that.

Our happiness tends to be based on a feeling attached to something—a situation, an outcome, an experience, or a fleeting moment. Happiness can be hard to maintain; it comes and goes similarly to how our emotions ebb and flow with our hormones. Joy, on the other hand, is steady and profound. It isn't based on any circumstance we're experiencing or not experiencing but is a state of *being*. Joy is based on a different formula and equation altogether.

Joy isn't just happiness; it's happiness with roots. The happiness we feel toward something good like a warm summer day or having a baby can't be compared to the joy and pleasure of knowing God. He is the creator of all goodness, joy, and happiness we experience.

Psalm 16:11 confirms that the Lord is our joy. "In your presence there is fullness of joy; at your right hand are pleasures forevermore" (ESV). Abundant pleasure is at the right hand of God, where Jesus sits in heaven. "I say to the LORD, 'You are my LORD; apart from you I have no good thing'" (Psalm 16:2). This verse declares that there is no good, no life, no happiness or joy apart from the Lord. He is the essence, creator, perfector, and giver of joy.

Please know that joy does not mean the absence of sadness or pain. Instead, the beauty of joy is that it remains even during the hardship and aches of life. For example, have you ever been to a funeral with someone who has experienced grief yet they are also at peace, somehow full of assurance in their sadness? This is a picture of real joy, not like the facade many of us put on, saying, "I'm fine; it's fine; everything's fine."

Only in Christ can we find complete joy. The shiny new car, perfect house, dream trip, or even the baby will never satisfy or be enough. John 15:11 describes overflowing joy like this: if we abide in Christ and keep his commandments, then his joy will be in us, and our joy will be full. The verses right beforehand give us the key to this overflowing joy: "I have loved you just as the Father has loved Me; remain in My love [and do not doubt My love for you]" (v. 9 AMP).

In Jesus' love for us, we can have joy that is complete and overflows.

An Invaluable Opportunity

I've seen how joy can be developed and gained during experiences when we are pulled and stretched, and our faith is needed. The Message version of James 1:3 says, "You know that under pressure, your faith-life is forced into the open and shows its true colors."

Thank you, James, for being so honest and direct to the early Christians, who were scattered due to hard times. In the Amplified version, the command in James 1:2–3 is translated as "Consider it nothing but joy, my brothers and sisters, whenever you fall into various trials. Be assured that the testing of your faith [through experience] produces endurance [leading to spiritual maturity, and inner peace]." James's goal was to get Christians to reevaluate the way we see trials.

Then in verse 4, he shared the reason: "Let endurance have its perfect result and do a thorough work, so that you may be perfect and completely developed [in your faith], lacking in nothing" (AMP). The Message version says, "Don't try to get out of anything prematurely. Let it do its work so you become mature and well-developed, not deficient in any way." As much as we fight it, it's okay to be in hard spaces; James said these difficulties are working in us.

Allow this trial to have its thorough work in you, knowing it will develop your faith. You're in the challenging process of maturing.

As Christians, we can view hardship and suffering differently. But how can we change this thinking in the middle of pain? First, hard times should not come as a surprise to us. James reminded us to consider it joy *whenever* we face trials—they were assumed because he knew we would face troubles. James knew we would need the inner peace and spiritual maturity that counting it all joy can lead to.

It's interesting that in Hebrew, *consider* means "to lead the way" or "turn over in one's mind,"[1] proving that our minds lead the way to pure joy and are an intricate and active part of our faith. Therefore, what we think shapes what we believe.

Once we recognize our hardship is not a curse and we are not victims, we can decide to shift our mindset toward rejoicing and believing that hardship is an opportunity. If we allow hard times to have their work in us, our perseverance will keep us from rushing out of them before God's willed timing for us. Instead, we are best developed through our trials, making us more complete and like Christ.

I understand this sounds impossible. However, I assume you are daily pleading for your fertility struggles to end. Like me, you've probably said something like, "Haven't I had enough yet, God? Can this be done, please?"

I implore you not to take your eyes off of the Lord, no matter how long it's been or how far you've walked away from him. He is never far, and you are never too far gone. Jesus is the author and perfecter of your faith (Hebrews 12:2). He will provide the perseverance you need.

Persevere in Christ

Trials may be the force, power, and driver for our joy. But "endurance produces character, and character produces hope" (Romans 5:4 ESV). Hope is our faith in Christ.

When we go through trials, we can persevere, meaning we resolve (decide in our mind) to do something despite difficulty or delay. Therefore, in the face of infertility, we can persevere in Christ. He is our example of an unswerving focus on God even as he suffered death on a cross. We find joy and peace in our waiting within his strength and comfort.

In 1 Peter 1:7–9, Peter told us that we could rejoice in our trials because they can have a significant purpose. He explained that trials help to prove that our faith is genuine, mature, and worth more than gold.

So even when the fire of infertility is refining you, know this: Jesus is making it worth more than gold in his eyes.

Reflect

- Do you believe God can give you joy even amid infertility? Why or why not?

_____

_____

_____

_____

_____

- How has waiting stretched your faith and matured you?

_____

_____

_____

_____

- What would it look like for you to persevere in this season? What would need to change?

_____

_____

_____

_____

_____

Pray

Lord God, I'm waiting for you. Even though I've had to suffer grief now, I know you're using each bit of it to grow my faith. May this painful journey result in my seeing more of you, praising you, and giving you more glory and honor. Though I can't understand what you are doing right now, may I trust you, love you, and believe in you, Father. Thank you that your presence fills me with unexplainable joy. You bring me hope, God, by who you are.

Act

Joy is found in our faith that God is working in us. Each day, challenge yourself to find one thing that brings you joy and write it on a sticky note. For example, take note of the sun shining on you, reminding you God created it to bring you warmth and light. Invite your husband to join you in doing this activity.

20

Desires of Your Heart

Delight yourself in the LORD, and he will
give you the desires of your heart.

Psalm 37:4 ESV

A bitter wind stung my mittenless hands. Despite the chill, I (Jenn) knocked at the door and waited for my friend Elizabeth to answer. Within seconds, she greeted me with a hug, balancing her two-year-old daughter on her hip, and hurried me into the warmth of her apartment.

We chatted while she heated water for tea. It wasn't until we sat down in her living room that she brought up the question I knew would come: "How are you doing?" I winced. My emotions were still raw after our failed IVF cycle, and I didn't feel like rehashing the devastation. Elizabeth waited patiently as I took another sip from my mug, stalling. Her daughter climbed in her lap, and Elizabeth began brushing her fingers through her toddler's tousled brown curls. Then the dam broke. I blurted, "I want God to take away my desire for a baby!"

Perhaps those words sound familiar to you. At some point on your journey, you might be done hoping. Your tears are spent, the pregnancy announcement gut punches keep coming, and you don't know how much longer you can live in limbo. If you're feeling this way, you're in good company. Throughout my years of infertility ministry, I've heard many women say they just want God to take away their desire for a baby.

I know what it's like to want your desire to disappear. You imagine life will be better if God would simply remove the source of your pain. But friend, I'm sorry to say, this prayer doesn't work. Asking God to take away the desire is really an attempt to avoid dealing with loss. We need to face our infertility grief, not try to escape it. Let me share three truths I discovered through my experience with unfulfilled desire.

A Child Is a Good Desire

From the beginning, we see that God delights in creating human life. First, he waited to call his creation "very good" until he formed Adam and Eve (Genesis 1:31). Then he told them to be fruitful and multiply—not as a promise of fertility but as an assignment to spread his kingdom throughout the world he made.

The creation story shows us that having a baby is God's idea. He came up with the process of conception, pregnancy, and birth. He's the master weaver who knits together tiny limbs within a mother's womb. Children are his heritage (Psalm 127:3), displaying his faithfulness from one generation to the next.

The Bible confirms that wanting a child is a good desire. Nowhere does it tell us we should pray for this desire to go away. You don't need to be ashamed of wanting to participate in God's beautiful design for nurturing life. He cares about your longing for a child and doesn't begrudge your desperate prayers.

God Is Our Greatest Desire

Like any desire, the desire for a child can take over all our other interests and activities. When we prioritize this one good desire above everything else, it can become the center of our lives to an unhealthy degree. Pastor Paul David Tripp explained how this happens: "The desire for even a good thing becomes a bad thing when that desire becomes a ruling thing."[1]

Our hearts can hold only one throne, and only God reserves the right to sit there. While wanting a child is a good desire, God created us to be fulfilled in *him*. Nothing else but God can satisfy our longings for joy, peace, purpose, wholeness, goodness, and no-strings-attached love.

Psalm 37:4 says, "Delight yourself in the LORD, and he will give you the desires of your heart" (ESV). This *doesn't* mean that if we love God, he'll give us whatever we want. God is our King, and we serve him, not the other way around. In this psalm, David wasn't talking about good desires we might request from God; he was declaring the goodness of running to God as our stronghold (Psalm 37:39).

God himself is the desire of our hearts. This is why, throughout Scripture, he urges us to seek him first (Matthew 6:33). We gain more fulfillment than we could hope for by delighting in him.

We Can Give Our Desire to Him

When we're feeling defeated, we might think our only options are wanting a baby too much or not wanting a baby at all. That's what I assumed, too, until the day I broke down at my friend's apartment.

After letting me vent, Elizabeth handed me a tissue, looked me square in the eyes, and said with gentle intensity, "I can understand why you'd feel that way. But Jenn, I don't think you should pray away the desire for a baby. God gave you that desire. Now give it over to him."

Give God my desire for a baby. I'd never thought of that before. My prayers usually consisted of pleading with God to fulfill my lifelong dream of being a mom. It hadn't occurred to me that instead of asking God to take away my desire, I could pray and ask him to *take care* of my desire.

Elizabeth pointed out an aspect of prayer that I'd missed. The Bible tells us to bring our requests to God in a specific way. "This is the confidence we have in approaching God: that if we ask anything *according to his will*, he hears us" (1 John 5:14, emphasis added). "According to his will" isn't just a phrase we tack on to the end of a prayer. This means we ask God to fulfill our desire for a child and also ask him to handle our desire the way he knows is best. As difficult as it is, we surrender our desire to the Lord.

I know surrendering your desire to God sounds like giving up. And even though you might have begged God to take away your desire, the truth is you're scared to let go of something so precious as the dream of cradling your baby in your arms.

But try to think about it the way my friend suggested. Surrender isn't giving up; it's giving over. God knows how much you ache for a child. He will work through your sorrow to bring his good purposes to pass. Remember, God wants us to desire him, which gives him glory and gives us the delight we crave.

Praying by faith in God's goodness can be painful, like prying your fingers loose from a tight fist. Yet surrendering your desire for a child frees you to accept unfathomable peace. Your loving Father will do what's right. His will is perfect, and you can trust him even when the trusting hurts.

Want What He Wants

Jesus gave us the ultimate example of what to do with unfulfilled desire. Before his arrest that led to the cross, he asked God to remove the cup of suffering that would be poured out on him. We can see the anguish as he resolved to give over his desire: "Father, if you are willing, take this cup from me; yet not my will, but yours be done" (Luke 22:42).

Here's your model for prayer. Though it's hard, you can surrender your desire to God because Jesus surrendered his life for you. If you know him, he lives in you and will empower you to say to God, "Your will be done."

With this confidence, go ahead and ask God to fulfill your desire for a child. Then ask him to help you want what he wants. He will help you entrust to him what's good—having a baby—and enjoy what's best—knowing him.

Reflect

- How do you feel about your desire for a child? Do you see your desire as good or as something to be removed?

_____

_____

_____

_____

- Has your desire for a child become the ruling desire of your heart? How? Be honest with God. When you admit that your desires are out of order, God can redirect your heart to seek fulfillment in him above everything else.

_____

_____

_____

_____

_____

- What's your gut reaction to the thought of surrender? Could you give over your desire for a child to the Lord right now? Or do you need to start by asking him to help you want to want his will?

_____

_____

_____

_____

_____

Pray

O Lord my God, you are worthy of all praise. The process you designed for growing life is wonderfully unbelievable. I know you can do anything, and *you hear my cries of longing. So I ask you to fulfill my desire and give me a baby. As I wait for your answer, help me entrust my desire to you. For you are my righteous King, the strength of my heart, and my portion forever (Psalm 73:26). As I surrender this good thing to you, please fill me with your all-satisfying love.*

Act

Open your hands in a visible act of surrender. Borrow Jesus' words from Luke 22:42, and say this prayer out loud: "Father, I give you my desire for a child. Not my will, Lord, but yours be done." If you need to, practice this daily. God can use this habit to bend your heart toward his.

LEANING
· ON ·
HOPE

✦

The Relational Journey

21

Love Your Beloved

The Lord God said, "It is not good for the man to be
alone. I will make a helper suitable for him."

Genesis 2:18

Roses, hydrangeas, and fresh, minty eucalyptus filled the air with romance.
It was a magical day. My heart leaped in anticipation of a future life wrapped
in his arms. Justin and I (Kelley) exchanged vows with tearful eyes and shak-
ing hands and promised to love, honor, and cherish each other.

From the beginning of our relationship, my husband and I committed
to putting the Lord's will and our marriage before everything else—other
relationships, work, opportunities, or trials that would come. But nothing
could prepare us for the nightmare of infertility and miscarriage. Unmet
expectations, strained finances, and overwhelming grief created friction
between us. When we tried to talk, it seemed that Justin no longer recognized me. To be honest, I'd become so consumed with wanting a baby that
I didn't recognize myself.

One awful night, I unleashed all my pent-up emotions on Justin, admitting that I'd been believing the lies of feeling crazy and ruined. (Side note:
crazy and *ruined* are words no longer allowed in our home.) Unsure how to

respond, he leaned in and whispered, "I miss my wife. I want her back." He was trying his best to keep our marriage afloat the primary way he knew how—by being strong and helping us survive. But with my hormones raging and my heart drowning in grief, all I could hear was, "My husband doesn't get me. I'm alone."

Husband + Wife = Family

Infertility, miscarriage, and waiting push our marriages into the "for worse," "in sickness," and "for poorer" parts of our vows. These daunting challenges can drive a bitter wedge between you and your husband. Perhaps you don't see eye to eye on fertility treatments. You might have different coping styles with stress, leading to a breakdown in communication. One or both of you might feel shame after receiving male- or female-factor diagnoses. Then there's the conflict if your husband isn't a Christian and doesn't share the same beliefs and values you hold dear.

I know how these struggles can rip apart your relationship with your husband. All the tension and arguments can wear you down and make you feel like you're losing the man you love.

Don't lose heart. God cares for your marriage, for you and your husband and your lives together. Remember that marriage was God's idea in the first place. Genesis 2:18 explains why he made man and woman: "The LORD God said, 'It is not good for the man to be alone. I will make a helper suitable for him.'" God didn't want Adam to be alone in humanity, so he created Eve to be his companion. The husband-wife relationship is so important that it's the first human bond God created.

Once God saw the universe he made, with man and woman as the crowning glory of his creation, he called it "very good" (Genesis 1:31). Notice that he said this before Eve got pregnant. In God's eyes, a husband and a wife are a family whether or not they have children.

Isn't it comforting to know you and your husband are already a family? Like any family, you support each other through the troubles of life. When one falls, the other lifts up. You sacrifice for the good of your relationship. For me, this looked like letting go of my desire to control our infertility journey and allowing my husband to lead us through making decisions. Having him take charge helped us face our struggles together instead of fighting against each other.

By making your husband part of this process, you can unite your family of two and show your husband you've got his back in the battle of waiting.

How to Reconnect with Your Husband

Marriage gives husbands and wives opportunities to love like Jesus. In our everyday moments, we can strengthen our relationship with each other and with the Lord, as author Gary Thomas pointed out in *Sacred Marriage*: "How can we use the challenges, joys, struggles, and celebrations of marriage to draw closer to God? What if God designed marriage to make us both happy and holy?"[1]

You and your husband can lead happy and holy lives as you wait for a child. However, it takes time, effort, and prayer to keep your relationship honest and close.

I know this might sound impossible. It did to me for a long time. You might feel like you've drifted so far away from your husband that you'll never be able to bridge the distance between you. With God's strength, you can do this. Just take one step at a time. Start with brainstorming ideas for how you can spend time together doing something you both enjoy. Go for walks with your dog, take a cooking class, play card games, or try an escape room together. Set a rule that you won't talk about anything baby-related during that time. Doing several of these dates will help you remember, *Yes! We really do like each other!*

After you've rekindled the joy you had before infertility, you and your husband can talk about family building with a united heart. You can share what you're feeling and remember that your husband has feelings too. Even when you're hurt by something he said or didn't say or angry with him for not understanding, take a deep breath and forgive him. Before you launch into a difficult conversation, ask the Holy Spirit to give you the patience to hear your husband's perspective and work with him to find solutions that benefit both of you.

If your husband doesn't know Jesus right now, having these conversations can be especially hard. Ask God to help you listen to his concerns and respond with gentleness and love. Keep praying for your husband to follow God and learn how to lead your family. If your husband can't offer spiritual guidance, you can turn to God's Word, trustworthy friends, counselors, and your local church for support and reminders of God's presence in your life, even now.

As you approach your husband with grace, believe that God can restore your marriage. No fractured relationship is beyond his healing power.

Choose Your Marriage

At some of the lowest points in our journey, my husband was quick to affirm his care for me. He said, "Kelley, I choose our marriage. I choose you over all of this, over a baby, and over your anger and sadness. Regardless of how this ends, we are a team." When I couldn't navigate the swirling chaos, I stayed anchored by my beloved's love.

You can choose your husband during this intense season. Invest in your relationship with him, remembering that you're already a family even before you welcome a child. If or when a baby comes, remember that you'll still need to make your husband a priority and set aside time for just the two of you.

You are your beloved's, and he is yours. Together, you can get through this season stronger than when you said, "I do."

Reflect

• What is your definition of *family*? How does the story of Adam and Eve affect your view of what it means to be a family?

_____

_____

_____

_____

_____

• How has infertility affected your relationship with your husband? In what ways might you need to apologize, clear up any misunderstanding, and/or seek restoration?

_____

_____

_____

_____

_____

- (*For the wife married to an unbeliever*) How can you show your husband love in a way that he may "be won" to faith (1 Peter 3:1)? Who are some godly people you can go to for support?

_____

_____

_____

_____

_____

Pray

Dear Father, the pain of infertility has come into every aspect of my life, including my relationship with my husband. We struggle to understand each other's emotions and often end up fighting whenever we talk about what we should or shouldn't do to have a baby. Lord, help restore our vision of your design for marriage. Repair the damage caused by the pressures of difficult circumstances and the consequences of our own mistakes. Reunite us through the perfect love of your Son, and motivate us to lay down our lives for him and for each other. We need your grace to bind us together.

Act

Plan a time with your husband to think about your wedding vows. Read them together and discuss the specific words you chose. Then repeat the vows out loud to each other.

If you don't feel comfortable asking your husband to join you, start by praying consistently and then waiting to see how God might work in your husband's heart. Consider talking to a pastor and/or counselor if the problems in your marriage are proving extremely difficult to resolve. Taking that step can be an act of courage to help you and your husband heal.

22

Redeeming the Bedroom

*That is why a man leaves his father and mother and
is united to his wife, and they become one flesh.*

Genesis 2:24

Tip: Read this chapter with your husband.

The clock was ticking, and we had precisely forty-five minutes. Which meant it was *go time!* Our doctor had dictated a schedule of twenty-four hours between times of intercourse, but our window was closing. Luckily, my husband was able to come home for a quick lunch break. But our plans were disrupted before they even began. The cable guy finally showed up—four hours late.

We couldn't kick him out, of course. Scrutinizing our lack of options, we knew this was our only chance. So we would have to go for it *quietly.*

I (Kelley) know we do some unusual things in this season of trying, especially when it comes to this integral and personal part of marriage. However, nothing is less romantic or intimate, and more stressful and mechanically forced, than a couples' sex life while trying to conceive.

Though this example may seem funny, it was what our sex life had become. We were no longer motivated by our love and enjoyment of each other, nor was sex even about us. We had put aside the true purpose of intimacy that we share with no one else.

Intimacy is rooted in who we are and attached to every aspect of our lives as a couple. Perhaps this is why problems we face in the bedroom can lead to further relational strains, sometimes becoming shockwaves felt for years to come. For example, one study indicated that couples who go through fertility treatment are up to three times more likely to divorce if they don't end up having a child.[1]

Most couples I've met share similar stories and difficulties, leading many to wonder, *Why isn't sex like it was before? Can it ever go back to the way it used to be?*

Kim explained the effects that trying to conceive had on her and her husband. She said, "Who wants to schedule sex? It feels so odd. I hated talking about it. So I started putting 'date night' on the calendar when I knew I was ovulating. For several months, we had to have sex three days in a row, so he knew that's what 'date night' signified."

Sex Is Much More

Intimacy and romance are inherently about our intimacy with God the Father. I know that can be a strange concept. But intimacy is the picture of us being fully seen, cared for, and loved, and is a crescendo display of God's unfathomable love for us.

In chapter 14, we discussed that the Enemy does not want you to have a relationship or intimacy with God. Therefore, Satan does not want you to have any joy of intimacy with your husband through the romance of sex.

But God desires much more for us. He created man and woman to be woven together. As literally "bone of my bones and flesh of my flesh" (Genesis

2:23), we are bonded and connected within marriage. Verse 24 commands us to leave our families and become physically and emotionally "one flesh" with our spouse. The Message version emphasizes this intimacy: "A man leaves his father and mother and embraces his wife. They become one flesh. The two of them, the Man and his Wife, were naked, but they felt no shame" (vv. 24–25).

God designed sex as a way to glorify himself and for us to enjoy the spouse he has given us. It is a gift granted to us for our delight and joy, as shown in Proverbs 5:18–19: "Rejoice in the wife of your youth. Let her breasts and tender embrace satisfy you. Let her love alone fill you with delight" (TLB).

Sex is an act of worship. When God created sex for Adam and Eve to enjoy within marriage, it was holy and pleasing. Our desire should be for our husband, and his desire should be for us. Yet like our biblical ancestors, we get distracted by the effects of the fall. Infertility is just another ripple effect of how the brokenness of sin creates friction and tries to destroy what God made for good and our pleasure.

First Corinthians 7 reminds us that in the marriage relationship, our bodies are not solely our own but yielded to our spouse, and sex is our marital duty. The Message version says, "It's good for a man to have a wife, and for a woman to have a husband. . . . The marriage bed must be a place of mutuality—the husband seeking to satisfy his wife, the wife seeking to satisfy her husband" (vv. 2–3).

As we endure pain in the pursuit of a baby, we can easily forget that God's design is for sex to be a delight and joy in each other, giving honor and glory to God.

Within marriage, sex is sacred. Our unity displays how much God loves us. Loving each other means yielding to each other, communicating openly, and expressing our love repeatedly.

Through the example of a loving marriage, we have the opportunity to represent Christ's unconditional love for both his church and for us.

Restoring the Joy of Intimacy

My husband and I were supposed to make a baby together through this loving act, but when we couldn't, I no longer wanted to have sex. So we were at a standstill, and it felt awful.

It's almost impossible for infertility not to impact our sex lives. But our marriages were not intended to be this way, and they do not have to remain how they've been.

Sex is the most personal and bonding aspect of our marriage, but the problem in my marriage came when we lacked the earnestness to discuss the real issues in detail. As a result, our bodies became worn down and separated—and so did our hearts.

If we brush this off as something that will get better on its own or solve itself later, we are setting ourselves up for further agony. With many couples, most issues or concerns in marriage become exacerbated and intensified in the season of infertility. Whether this is relational, financial, or emotional—whatever it may be for you in your marriage—if ignored, the issue will eventually spill over into more areas of your life.

Understandably, we can become so invested in our fertility hopes that our intimacy is hijacked by trying to conceive. But when sex becomes a means to an end and more important than being with and enjoying your spouse, maybe it's time to pause and refocus.

- *Openly talk about sex together.* Discuss with your spouse the specific issues, preferences, and needs before they grow into greater resentment, discontentment, or bitterness. Remember, husbands can't read our minds. We shouldn't expect them to know what we need or want. Share with him your expectations of how he can help you.
- *Make sex fun again.* Remember what sex was like before infertility. Be

spontaneous, playful, flirty, and make efforts for it to be important again.

- *Initiate intimacy.* My husband once said to me, "I'd like you to initiate intimacy during unexpected and not required times, so I don't feel like a sperm donor. So it's about just me and not about what I can possibly provide for us." Approach your husband for intimacy during times when it's not about having a baby.
- *Work to keep your marital bed God-honoring.* Consider putting safeguards in place to honor your union and oneness. For instance, Justin and I decided early on that anything surrounding "making a baby" needed to include only the two of us and adhere to the Spirit's convictions for both of us:
  - With medical help, we tried to keep physical intimacy key. For example, I always helped with sperm samples to keep it about us.
  - If told to abstain from sex or take birth control, we prayed about it and decided together whether this would be best for us in the current phase before heeding the doctors' orders.
  - We prayed before and after sex, praising God and thanking him for our union and protection.

Consider how you can allow God to redeem, protect, and provide for your sexual oneness. I've walked with others whose marriages were fractured, but God revitalized them in his beautiful grace.

A Redemptive Place

Joy can abound in our enjoyment of each other. Sex is not meant to be a chore or only what we do to make a baby or bring pleasure to our spouse.

It's a consummation of God's beauty in marriage that we are seen for who we are, naked and unashamed (Genesis 2:25).

Nothing is beyond the redeeming and healing hands of Jesus' grace and redemptive work on the cross, not even our disconnected sex life. His redemptive work can occur within the intimate nuances, tenderness, and compassionate aspects of the bedroom.

I encourage you to be brave enough to open your heart in vulnerability with your spouse. Allowing Christ's love to pour out of you and onto your spouse can improve your marriage. As my friend Kasey shared, "Sex became mainly about timing for me, and I became very emotional during intimacy. God helped restore the joy of our intimacy when I began to see it as a gift, not as a means to an end."

Reflect

- How has infertility affected your intimacy in marriage? Write down what sex was like in the past, how it is now, and how you'd like it to be different.

_____

_____

_____

_____

_____

- How could you adjust or place safeguards in trying to conceive, to put God and each other first?

_____

_____

_____

_____

_____

• Do you believe God can redeem your intimacy and make your bedroom a loving, enjoyable space again? If God can create from nothing, if Jesus can heal people and rise from the grave, then he can restore what infertility has damaged.

_____

_____

_____

_____

_____

Pray

Heavenly Father, begin to stir in my heart and my husband's heart a new desire for you and a deeper love for each other through our love for you. As we look to you, Lord, draw us closer as only you can do. Redeem our intimacy and union with each other to be a holy act of surrender. Make us whole together as one flesh. Remove any obstacle, dissension, or barrier the Enemy uses in an attempt to wedge us apart. Instead, make our desire stronger for you and for each other. May we long for a marriage and intimacy that are new again.

Act

Discuss this chapter's Reflect questions with your husband. Then spend time on your bed, admiring each other, your bodies, hearts, and whole persons, and allow for enjoyment and fun. Make sex romantic and flirty in the way it used to be before this season. Yes, sex is our marital duty to give our bodies over to our spouse, for our bodies are not our own (1 Corinthians 7:4–5), but sex should be a delight.

The Bible does not give our spouses permission to assert dominance over us, and it does not permit them to appease their sexual desires in ways other than the marital union. Instead, it shows just how connected our bodies and sex are to the Father. If you are experiencing abuse or circumstances you are uncomfortable with in your marriage, do not delay in removing yourself from the situation, then seek immediate help and counseling.

23

One Happy Family

Be kind and compassionate to one another, forgiving
each other, just as in Christ God forgave you.

Ephesians 4:32

"When are you going to have kids?" We hear it at every holiday gathering, birthday party, and family reunion. This question always seems to put us on the spot at the exact moment when the entire family is listening. How are we supposed to answer without bawling in front of everyone?

Family relationships are tough to manage during infertility. Because our family members are often the people closest to us, they have the greatest potential to wound us, whether they intend to or not. Maybe you can relate to what some of our Waiting in Hope Chats members have experienced:[1]

- Nagging about giving your parents or in-laws a grandchild.
- Criticism of your decision to skip family gatherings.
- Unwanted opinions about when you should see a doctor, which fertility treatments you should or shouldn't do, and if you should pursue adoption.

- Judgment for seeing a doctor, trying fertility treatments, or adopting instead of trusting God.

Infertility makes complicated family dynamics even trickier. Julie, a member of our Waiting in Hope community, felt an amped-up tension with her in-laws. They didn't approve of their son marrying her because Julie and her husband are an interracial couple. So when they tried to get pregnant and realized it wouldn't be easy, they hesitated to share their fertility struggles with her in-laws.

"We didn't want to hear a lecture of, 'Well, if you had listened to us' or 'This is what you get for marrying interracially,'" Julie said. "We knew they would see our infertility as an opportunity to say, 'I told you so.'"

While I (Jenn) don't know your unique family situation, I'm willing to guess one or more relatives have hurt you. These are the people who are supposed to have our backs when life bullies us around. So when they give us dismissive words instead of shoulders to cry on, it feels like betrayal.

How to Respond

As much as our families can add to our pain, we need to recognize that their insensitivity usually comes from ignorance, not cruelty. For most of us, our family members haven't been through infertility. They have no idea what an IUI is, how much adoption costs, or why we can't just move on after suffering miscarriage.

As you struggle with family members who don't understand you, remember God knows your grief better than anyone. He meets you in your pain and offers his protection as your shield and strength. Take heart in David's words in Psalm 27:10: "Even if my father and mother abandon me, the LORD cares for me" (CSB). God cares for you, his beloved daughter. Your family might insult you, forget your miscarried baby's due date, or make you dread spending time together. But you can count on your Father to stay with you every step of your journey.

As God's children, we are representatives of his Son. Representing Jesus involves following his example in our thoughts, words, desires, and actions. Our waiting season gives us the opportunity to show our families who Jesus is. Though they hurt us, in his strength we can treat our relatives the way Jesus interacted with people. This means instead of snapping at them, we respond with kindness. Instead of harboring resentment, we consider how to meet their needs. Instead of raging against their opinions, we forgive them.

Forgiving your family might sound impossible to you. That makes sense because it *is* impossible. We can't forgive others in our own strength. Thankfully, we don't have to.

Ephesians 4:32 says, "Be kind and compassionate to one another, forgiving each other, just as *in Christ* God forgave you." God didn't forgive our sins based on our works. He forgave us because Jesus paid the debt we could never afford. Just as he canceled our wrongs, he'll one day correct all the wrongs committed against us.

You don't have to carry the wrongs done to you by your family. Jesus already carried them for you. *In Christ*, you can forgive them. Not because you feel guilty or because your family deserves it—they might not. It's the power of Christ living in you that gives you courage to do the impossible.

Steps for Better Relationships

Forgiving others doesn't make you a doormat. You can take the initiative to improve relationships with family members for your benefit and theirs.

Here are a few suggestions:

- *Acknowledge the hurt.* First, bring your pain to the Lord. As he works his healing in your life, talk to the family member who hurt you. Be honest and specific. Gently explain why their comment added to your pain. Then offer ideas for what they could say instead.
- *Ask the Spirit to help you with self-control.* Let's be honest—we're not our best selves when dealing with runaway hormones and grief. Pray that the Holy Spirit will give you strength to rein in your temper and wisdom to know when to speak and when to let things go.
- *Prepare yourself.* It's almost guaranteed that some family member will ask awkward questions when you least expect it. Better to have a go-to answer than fumble for words in the heat of embarrassment. At Waiting in Hope, we call this your "elevator pitch"—a twenty- to sixty-second prepared response that gives you confidence to answer the way you'd prefer.
- *Pray for a tender heart.* Julie wanted to avoid her in-laws because of their constant lectures. Prayer was the main thing that helped her respond with grace. She said, "The Holy Spirit gave me eyes to see that their questions and comments were out of ignorance. I had to realize there was nothing I could do to change anyone's mind or heart in regard to infertility, adoption, or anything else." The same is true for you. Before asking God to change your family's hearts, start with asking him to soften yours.

Forgiveness for Cluelessness

Right before his final breath, Jesus uttered a prayer for those who nailed him to the cross: "Father, forgive them, for they do not know what they are doing" (Luke 23:34). Your family is probably clueless about infertility. When it comes to supporting you, they likely have no idea what they're doing. Even if they make judgmental comments intentionally, you can ask the Father to forgive them. Because Jesus forgave those who killed him, you can forgive too.

Who knows? God might use this complicated time to bring you and your family closer together. But regardless of what happens with them, you can trust God will use your waiting season to draw you closer to him.

Reflect

- How have your family members reacted to your fertility struggles? If they've hurt you, take time to process what they said or did and why it hit you so hard.

_____

_____

_____

_____

_____

- In what ways have you responded to your family's reactions? Consider how you might have treated them unkindly, and come up with ideas for different ways of responding to them next time.

_____

_____

_____

_____

_____

- How can you use your waiting season to represent Christ to your family?

_____

_____

_____

_____

_____

Pray

Dear Jesus, I'm at a loss for how to approach my family. Rather than encourage me through this ordeal, they've made the journey more difficult. I come before you, laying down all the ways they've been insensitive toward me. Help change my attitude, doing your holy work of growing the fruit of compassion, kindness, and forgiveness. Thank you for paying the debt for my wrongs and theirs. Redeem my family drama as you've redeemed my life.

Act

Write down the first initial(s) of the family member(s) who hurt you. Now pray through forgiveness for each of them and ask the Lord to soften your heart toward them.

Create your elevator pitch for the question, "When are you going to have kids?" You'll be glad you have this prepared during difficult conversations.

If you're still struggling with deep wounds inflicted by family members or difficult family circumstances, consult a trusted counselor or therapist to discuss your emotions and setting healthy boundaries.

Friends Again

Dear friends, since God so loved us, we
also ought to love one another.

1 John 4:11

We were both pulling away from each other. I (Kelley) could sense it. After years of friendship, we now had little to no shared experiences together. We had laughed, cried, and guessed our way through the first few years of marriage and careers. But this felt so much harder than anything we had experienced before.

I didn't know how to talk about my infertility, and I worried about becoming a broken record she couldn't listen to anymore. Meanwhile, she didn't know what to say, what not to say, how to say it, or how to be pregnant around me. Deep down, she felt awful and guilty for having what she had. Though I felt sad and disappointed, I was really grieving over my desperate desire to be where she was, together.

We were worlds apart, and I wondered whether we would ever get back to "us" again. I began to question if our friendship would suffer or disappear and how we could ever make it through this pain. Could we be friends again?

We all experience pain in our friendships during this season, and sometimes these hurt the worst. Our friends should be for us and with us, but instead, it can seem like they are on another team altogether. Have your friendships become distant and more challenging, leaving you wondering what to do and how they will recover?

That's difficult to answer because friendship can have its challenges in any season. However, I have learned that friendships can actually become better when you both put in the important effort to be loving friends.

Tone Down Expectations

My friend and I didn't restore our friendship overnight. However, though it required our taking sensitive and healthy steps toward each other, it was possible.

First, I began to realize that my friend and I had come to this new season with unmet expectations that things would stay the same. This, combined with the fact that we weren't expressing our feelings, caused tension.

We often set expectations for friends and end up disappointed because only Jesus can meet our high standards of care. It's human nature to feel hurt and be wounded by others, because we're emotional beings and humans will never be perfect. As a result, we continually sin against each other, choose selfishness, and lack the all-knowing understanding to do the right thing at the right time.

My friendship started struggling when I refused to reach out to my friend, engage with her, or even care for her because of my own hurt, broken, and sinful places. Even though, deep down, I cared intensely for her, the ugliness of infertility pain had turned me inward instead of outward.

We tend to think our friends should understand because they know us. But how could they? Unless they have been in our shoes or walked the path of infertility, there's no way they can fully understand these aches.

Our friends' inability to relate isn't their fault, just like our inability to sympathize with their discomforts in motherhood is not our fault. Perhaps we've forgotten that our friends have hard times and frustrations or might be struggling with similar issues in a different context. Fear, loneliness, and hormonal upheavals could be our shared experiences right now. In 1 Peter 3:8, Peter said that every Christian believer is called to obey these five commands in relationships: "Finally, all of you, be like-minded, be sympathetic, love one another, be compassionate and humble." As hard as it might be, we can demonstrate these traits in our friendships.

If this seems too difficult, simply start by asking God to help you love your friend. Praying for someone inevitably softens your heart toward them, and over time, God's heart will become yours. As we pray, we can see our friends correctly as broken people doing their best.

When we no longer expect our friends to meet our needs, we can take our needs to Jesus, who can satisfy every longing and fill us. We no longer need to be validated or demand love from others when we are in his care.

Address the Elephant in the Room

No one wants to be the person to initiate the hard conversations, or at least I don't. Yet I've learned that stepping into the hard places is necessary and a God-glorifying opportunity. I now firmly believe that there is a reason from God if I'm the one to notice an issue. It's typically been the areas or people I've wanted to avoid that God wants me to deal with the most.

So let's look at some potential steps to address the elephant in the room you've been avoiding in your friendships.

- *Start the conversation.* Share that you value your friendship too much to see this season get between you, and you want to continue investing and enjoying time together.

- *Say "I'm sorry."* Admit that you've been upset. Say something like, "It's not your fault that you are pregnant or a mom, and I'm not."
- *Share how it made you feel.* Try to use "I feel" statements; this is easier for others to receive. Be honest. Share how platitudes and unsolicited advice can worsen your hurt.
- *Suggest ways she can help.* Tell your friend specific ways to help care for you. If she asks this in the conversation, she's amazing! If not, consider letting her know this book has a section just for her called "Help Me Wait."
- *Return the favor.* Be a good, responsive friend by asking her what you could do to help her in your friendship, then listen and receive what she says.
- *Give her time to process.* Be patient; it may take her time even after you've talked. Put aside your defenses, remembering this is a challenging and tricky conversation she probably wasn't ready to hear. Patience is a two-way street that moves us toward healing. Approach her with humility and out of love, as Paul encouraged us in Ephesians 4:2 and Philippians 2:3.
- *Set healthy and loving boundaries.* Pray about whether to accept invitations to baby showers, dedications, birthday parties, or girls' nights out. If any environment will threaten your emotional or spiritual state, you might be better off declining graciously. Explain why it's too hard to go, reminding others it's not about them but the pain of the circumstances. Then be the fun friend who shows up another time to celebrate.

Vulnerability creates vulnerability. Therefore, the more honest you are with your friend, the better. Even in your vastly different phases, you can both be loved as you look to the Father, who will make you more like Jesus.

Live at Peace

The friendship I discussed earlier required real heart work to get to the place of being close friends again. It took a lot of grace and forgiveness on both our parts.

Romans 12:18 says, "If it is possible, as far as it depends on you, live at peace with everyone." If you have prayed and sought the Lord in handling this friendship, you have done what you can. Even when friendships don't heal, trust that God knows what this friendship meant, and he hasn't forgotten you.

I've heard that friends come into our lives for a season, for a reason, or for a lifetime. Continue to respond to your friend in love, knowing it's ultimately her choice how to move forward. Regardless, you can know you did your part to bring about Jesus' peace. He is your most faithful friend.

Reflect

- Do you have a hypersensitive attitude toward your friends? Be honest. Your emotions are valid and often hard to face. But through Jesus, you can take ownership of your actions.

_____

_____

_____

_____

_____

- Whom do you need to forgive? Whom do you need to ask for forgiveness?

_____

_____

_____

_____

_____

- In what ways can you extend grace to your friend? Instead of expecting your friends to say something hurtful, look for whatever is good, true, lovely, and worthy of praise (Philippians 4:8).

_____

_____

_____

_____

_____

Pray

Lord Jesus, I come to you saddened by the change in my friendship. Help me to own my part in the separation between us and aim for peace and harmony, for the sake of the gospel and my heart. Will you enter this place between my friend and me and heal what has been broken? Enable us to communicate *openly and trust each other again. If this friendship is not what you'd have for me, then allow me to see that. Lord, you are more worthy than any earthly friendship.*

Act

Plan a coffee date (or whatever fun thing you like to do together) with your friend to reconnect. Tell your husband your plan of action or the next right step with this friendship.

25

Sharing the Comfort

Praise be to the God and Father of our Lord Jesus Christ,
the Father of compassion and the God of all comfort, who
comforts us in all our troubles, so that we can comfort those in
any trouble with the comfort we ourselves receive from God.

2 Corinthians 1:3–4

My waiting season took a U-turn the day I (Jenn) met Don and Pam. Our paths crossed at an adoption seminar where the married couple shared their story. When they were going through the adoption process, God gave them the idea to start an infertility support group. What began as a handful of people gathered at their church eventually grew into a citywide ministry.

As Don and Pam spoke, I heard the passion in their voices. It was clear that leading the support group had given them purpose in their struggles. When the seminar ended, I jumped out of my seat and bombarded them with questions. I was eager to learn more about this ministry that blessed them as they linked arms with other couples trying to grow their families.

For the first time in two-and-a-half years, I felt a spark of hope. Finally, here was something I could *do* with my grief. The thought of helping people brought exciting possibilities. If God could use Don and Pam to encourage those hurting, maybe he could use me too.

The Invitation in Our Pain

When I began struggling with infertility, I shut out other people for self-protection. My focus shrank to what I didn't have and how I could avoid more pain. God gradually revived me by lifting my eyes from myself to those around me.

I remember how hard it is to look past your tears. Though your hurt feels personal, I can assure you your infertility isn't just about you. One way God gives purpose to our pain is by working through us to comfort others. Paul explained this in 2 Corinthians 1:3–4: "Praise be to the God and Father of our Lord Jesus Christ, the Father of compassion and the God of all comfort, who comforts us in all our troubles, so that we can comfort those in any trouble with the comfort we ourselves receive from God."

The God of all comfort doesn't leave us to ache alone. Instead, our Father draws close to us with compassion, applying his mercies like balm on our wounds. As God comforts us, he wants us to pass the comfort to others. We receive so we can give.

Paul received this kind of comfort in all types of affliction. He was beaten, imprisoned, stoned, shipwrecked, and almost starved. Throughout his near-death experiences, Paul believed his suffering was for the sake of God's people. "If we are distressed, it is for *your* comfort and salvation; if we are comforted, it is for *your* comfort, which produces in you patient endurance of the same sufferings we suffer" (2 Corinthians 1:6, emphasis added).

If we're beaten down by infertility, we know God will use it for someone else's benefit. It's not through our strength but through our suffering that others see the hope of Christ. I love how Ann Voskamp described our calling in brokenness: "He's inviting me to heal, but also to see my most meaningful calling: to be his healing to the hurting. My own brokenness, driving me into Christ's, is exactly where I can touch the brokenhearted."[1]

This is God's invitation to you. He says, *Come to my Son, who was broken for you. As you receive comfort from him, your brokenness will become my instrument of mercy to others.*

Empowered by the Spirit

At this point you might be thinking, *Being God's instrument sounds nice. But how can I help anyone right now? I'm in the middle of my wait, barely surviving each day. How am I supposed to offer comfort to others when I'm a mess?*

The first thing I suggest is to acknowledge reality. You're a mess. So am I. We can start a new-mercy-needing, not-so-hot-mess club together. Both of us depend on God's grace every moment of every day. Remember, the comfort we share isn't our own. We have the Spirit of God living in us. Our Helper gives us comfort, wisdom, and courage to follow Christ. And we know one of the main ways to follow Christ is to tell others about him. In his last minutes on earth, Jesus told his disciples why they were about to receive the Spirit's power: to be his witnesses (Acts 1:8).

If you've committed your life to Jesus, you have this same power inside you. Rely on the Spirit to help you be a witness to a hope-hungry world.

Here are a few practical ideas for sharing comfort through the Spirit's strength.

- *Look around you.* God is the King of details. He placed you where you are, at a time when you're struggling, for specific reasons (Acts 17:26).

Someone in your life needs a lifeline. You could be the person who introduces them to Jesus. Ask the Lord to give you eyes to notice what my grandmother called "divine appointments."

- *Weep together.* The comfort of Christ goes beyond feeling bad for someone. Our gentle and lowly Savior listened with compassion and offered the kindness of his touch. By following Jesus' example, you can give people the gift of a quiet companion to join in their weeping.
- *Use your gifts.* Believe it or not, you're gifted. God designed you with unique talents and interests to share with others. For example, if you're good at hand-lettering, you could make someone a print of a Bible verse. Or if you've got a knack for numbers, offer your budget-planning services. Whatever your hands find to cook, paint, organize, repair, or decorate, do it to glorify God by serving others.
- *Step out of your comfort zone.* Your pain could be someone else's path to Christ. But for them to see the hope, you have to do the hard work of vulnerability. There are many ways you can share your journey online and in person. However, this doesn't mean spilling everything on social media, unless God leads you in that direction. Also, don't forget the old-fashioned practice of striking up a conversation with a neighbor, coworker, or the woman sitting next to you at the fertility clinic waiting room.

Hope, Multiplied

After talking to Don and Pam, I met with one of the pastors at my church to ask about starting an infertility support group. To my surprise, he told me another woman had just brought up the same idea. That woman became my dear friend and coleader of the first infertility support group in our community. Her name is Kelly.

Eight years later, the Holy Spirit nudged me to form an online community for encouragement during infertility. As I was doing research, I came across a ministry that offered in-person and online support groups. The founder and I messaged back and forth, praying and dreaming of what God could do through us working together. You know her as my coauthor of this book, Kelley—cofounder (with her husband, Justin) of Waiting in Hope Ministries.

This is what happens when you become God's broken instrument. You get to watch the Spirit move in ways only he can orchestrate.

Wherever you are on your journey, you can be sure God will place opportunities for you to help others. Trust me, you'll be blessed if you take them. Serve the hurting people you meet. Give from the reserve you don't think you have, which comes from the Spirit dwelling within you. He'll help you be someone's Don and Pam.

Reflect

• Do you struggle with wanting to isolate yourself from other people? What motivates you to consider others' needs and hurts?

_____

_____

_____

_____

_____

- Is it easy or difficult to believe your infertility could provide an opportunity to comfort someone?

_____

_____

_____

_____

_____

- Does sharing the good news of Jesus sound intimidating to you? How can you remind yourself that the Holy Spirit will give you the courage to show your wounds?

_____

_____

_____

_____

_____

Pray

God of my comfort, I thank you for pouring your mercy on me. I confess infertility has put blinders on me, turning my focus away from other people. Please stir my heart with deep compassion for those who are suffering. Help *me look for people who could use encouragement from someone who knows pain. Give me the courage to be bold, and make me your broken instrument of life-saving hope.*

Act

Pick one person in your life who is in pain (infertility or not), and seek an opportunity to comfort them.

If you don't have a community to share your journey, check out the Waiting in Hope Ministries website (waitinginhopeinfertility.com) and join the online group or in-person groups. Or consider this a nudge from God to start a support group in your community. We have resources to help!

WALKING

·WITH·

HOPE

✦

Journeying Forward

26

Should We Do IVF? (and Other Decisions)

Trust in the LORD with all your heart and lean not
on your own understanding; in all your ways submit
to him, and he will make your paths straight.

Proverbs 3:5–6

No one can prepare for the kind of news the doctor gave Lauren and her husband: "You'll never conceive naturally." After years of disappointment and several failed IUIs, they had held on to hope for a miracle from God. Yet here they were, hearing that their next and final step had to be IVF. With this major crossroads before them, the couple took time to consider how IVF would fit with their faith and convictions.

During this process, Lauren felt the burden of such a complex decision. "These conversations and decisions are nuanced and incredibly weighty," she said. "Honestly, I think however anyone chooses to walk through infertility is good, as long as they are seeking to remain faithful to their convictions and obedient to the Lord."

As we walk through infertility, our journeys branch in many hazy directions. Each way requires a decision that could change our lives forever:

Should we get another opinion?
Should we take a break?
Should we look into adoption?
Should we do IVF?
Should we quit?

Though the way forward is daunting, you can take courage. God is bigger than all the big decisions you have to make. Look at what Moses told Joshua and the Israelites before they entered the promised land: "The LORD himself goes before you and will be with you; he will never leave you nor forsake you. Do not be afraid; do not be discouraged" (Deuteronomy 31:8). Just as the Lord faithfully led his people through the wilderness, he will go before you on the dark, winding paths of infertility.

Like Lauren, you can weigh your options in a way that honors God and your convictions. It starts with what you choose to seek.

Answers Versus Wisdom

When my husband and I (Jenn) were facing decisions about IVF and adoption, I wanted God to give us clear directions. A road map, a neon sign, a burning bush—any method of communication would have been helpful. To me, seeking his will meant looking for answers.

What about you? Are you also wishing for a sign from God? You might have flipped to this chapter hoping Kelley or I would tell you a straight yes or no about trying IVF.

It's true that *sometimes* God nudges us toward a specific path he wants us to take. But he doesn't reveal everything about his plans. The Lord's hidden will belongs to him alone (Deuteronomy 29:29). This is hard to accept when we're desperate to know how to have a child. Yet God is still God whether or not we hear him say, *This is the way.* He has good plans for us, plus good reasons for how, when, and if he reveals them to us.

If God gave us all the answers, we wouldn't need to trust him. Instead, he wants us to lean on him, not our own understanding. Proverbs 2:6 says, "For the LORD gives wisdom; from his mouth come knowledge and understanding."

God's wisdom is revealed in more than his answering questions about what we should do. Charles Haddon Spurgeon explained the distinction: "Wisdom is better than knowledge, for wisdom is knowledge rightly used. Knowledge may find room for folly, but wisdom casts it out. Knowledge may be the horse, but wisdom is the driver. . . . We want Christian people not only to know, but to use what they know."[1]

Seeking wisdom isn't simply a matter of asking the Lord, "Should I turn left here?" To receive wisdom, we seek the Lord himself. We believe in his sovereignty, obey his commands, and follow his Spirit's promptings as we make choices and walk by faith.

Tools for Gaining Wisdom

As you seek God on your journey, you can find his wisdom if you know where to look. Let's look at three tools he provides that can shed light on your decisions about how to resolve infertility.

The Wisdom of God's Word

Maybe you're familiar with this often-quoted verse: "Your word is a lamp for my feet, a light on my path" (Psalm 119:105). Notice the lamp is for our feet. It doesn't shine on everything around or in front of us. God's Word provides just enough light to help us take one step forward.

Obviously, the Bible doesn't mention IVF or assisted reproductive technologies.[2] It doesn't state a universal command about how everyone should address their childlessness. Instead, God's Word equips us for every good work (2 Timothy 3:16). The treasury of his wisdom offers principles for how we can love God, love people, and expand his kingdom.

Though the Bible doesn't explicitly address modern medical technologies or interventions, you can still search for truths and apply them to your decisions. For example, after studying Scripture, Lauren and her husband came to regard each embryo as a child. Their conviction to give every embryo a chance at life in their family led them to choose mini-IVF as the best option for their situation.

Whether or not you're considering IVF, the Bible will be your compass through infertility. If you dive into Scripture to grow closer to Jesus—not just to find answers about fertility issues—God will renew your mind (Romans 12:2). You can use this new, Christlike way of thinking to help discern which path to take.

The Wisdom of Prayer

You might think it sounds too easy to be true: "If any of you lacks wisdom, you should ask God, who gives generously to all without finding fault, and it will be given to you" (James 1:5). To get wisdom, all we have to do is ask.

God cares about *what* we ask for, as well as *how* we ask. He tells us to ask by faith, with humility, according to his will (Matthew 21:22; 2 Chronicles 7:14; 1 John 5:14). We commit our ways to him, acknowledging his authority over medicine, doctors, adoption agencies, and our bodies.

Prayer isn't a transaction; it's a means of transformation. As we pray, God repositions our hearts away from our self-centeredness and toward him. Then we surrender and say, "Amen," which means, "So be it, God." We place our desire back in God's hands and trust his will.

Of course, our prayers should go beyond asking for wisdom about fertility decisions. We need the Holy Spirit to guide us in truth, including the truth about our motives. Are we trying to control our circumstances or looking for comfort in the wrong places? He can lead us in making sound decisions for the right reasons.

The Wisdom of Godly Counsel

No one gets me. This is one of the loudest lies that taunts us during infertility. Don't believe it for a minute. Many other women and men have walked this road before you. While I was waiting, I learned from mentors who understood my grief because they'd lived it. These trusted friends kept me grounded in faith through their advice and example.

God's wisdom runs through the body of Christ—all those who believe in his Son. We can learn from other Christians who have struggled with infertility. Their experiences and decisions offer us an invaluable resource.

Proverbs 13:20 says, "Walk with the wise and become wise, for a companion of fools suffers harm." In this age of social media, we need to be selective about who we take with us on this journey. The most trustworthy counsel comes from people who defer to the Bible as the ultimate source of truth.

It's wise to seek input from friends, family, pastors, and other spiritual leaders. Just make sure to hold up God's Word as a filter to their advice.

Submit Your Ways to Him

If all this wisdom talk sounds overwhelming, that's because the options for addressing infertility *are* overwhelming. Take comfort knowing the Lord establishes your steps (Proverbs 16:9). Trusting him is an ongoing process that lasts through this season and beyond.

Ease up on the pressure on yourself. Making wise decisions about infertility doesn't come down to choosing the "right" path. The point is to submit your whole journey to the Lord. As Lauren said, "It's a continual act of reorienting, repenting, and refocusing on who is in control and what his heart is toward me."

Reflect

- When you pray about fertility decisions, what are you expecting from God? Are you pursuing his wisdom or hoping for a direct, "burning bush"–style answer about what you should do? (Read Exodus 3 for the story of how God called Moses through a burning bush.)

_____

_____

_____

_____

_____

- Which tools have you used to gain wisdom? Is one tool more difficult than another for you to apply? If so, jot down ideas for how you can start tapping into that resource.

_____

_____

_____

_____

_____

- How are you trusting God with your decision-making? This *doesn't* mean that choosing to go through fertility testing or treatment shows you lack faith. To walk through infertility by faith, we pray for wisdom, discern the most God-honoring option before us, and then take the next step, surrendering the outcome to him.

_____

_____

_____

_____

_____

Pray

Lord God, you are sovereign over all things, including all paths for addressing infertility. I admit, just looking at the options is exhausting. It would be so much easier if you'd tell me what to do. I need you to shift my desires from seeking answers to seeking your face. Please grant me wisdom to think through the options. Renew my mind so I can discern choices that conform to your Word. I don't know where you're leading me, but I trust you.

Act

Go on a prayer walk with your husband. Ask God to direct your steps and tell him you're actively placing your trust in him.

IVF and all assisted reproductive technologies are medical interventions. As authors, we aren't qualified to provide medical diagnoses or recommendations. These procedures entail many complex physiological and ethical implications that can't be covered within the scope of this book. We encourage you to seek medical advice from qualified medical professionals.

27

At What Cost?

*What is more, I consider everything a loss because
of the surpassing worth of knowing Christ Jesus
my Lord, for whose sake I have lost all things.*

Philippians 3:8

Some of the toughest questions in life revolve around money.

Should we pay to get our kitchen remodeled?
Is it time for a new car?
Should we give to that need or save up for our dream?

Of course, costs come in different forms. You discover this quickly when
you start going to the doctor for fertility tests. Not only do you have to fork
over a fortune, but you also take on heavy costs within yourself.

Our struggles weigh heavily not only within our hearts but also on those
around us. Our relationships—husbands, friends, coworkers, neighbors—
bear the burden as well. After you've expended so much, the toll eventually
catches up to you.

"We learned the hard way that once a miracle baby is in your arms, the marriage problems, financial struggles from multiple IVFs, anger at God, and broken friendships don't all heal or go away," said Brandy, a Waiting in Hope support group leader. "On the other side of our journey, we had to deal with the brokenness while also trying to navigate parenthood."

Remember that whatever the cost, the Lord is all-powerful. He controls everything that confuses you. God knew you'd be here, has a plan for this, and will fully prepare you even if you don't realize it yet.

Jesus paid the highest cost of all so that we wouldn't have our sins counted against us. By carrying our greatest burden for us, Jesus set us free from the penalty of sin. And he can still carry you through the costly process of waiting.

Dear friend, in this chapter I (Kelley) will ask you to take a hard look at your life, heart, and surroundings. Then seek the Lord's wisdom as you count the costs.

The Burden on Our Bodies

Infertility depletes us in a hundred different ways. Our bodies go through wild changes weekly, daily, and sometimes hourly. We aren't prepared for the fatigue, bruises, insomnia, weight gain, or bloating from fertility treatments.

The physical toll can make you lose motivation to take care of your body, put in quality work at your job, and engage in your favorite activities. Then there's the problem of how infertility lowers your sex drive.

During my journey, you could tell I was struggling by the wear and tear on my body. At other times, the emotional strain proved to be more intense. I think of it like an iceberg: one-third is above the water, while the majority is underwater. For a ship, the greater danger is the ice the captain can't see.

Like the iceberg, I appeared fine on the surface until I wasn't. In a split second, all the disappointment, fear, grief, and other emotions would turn into an erupting volcano. I'd find myself thinking, *Oops, I didn't know all that was there!*

The pain we experience in infertility can become unresolved pain. Richard Rohr explained how this happens: "If we do not transform our pain, we will most assuredly transmit it."[1]

You can't avoid pain in life. Yet you can learn to address it by looking to Jesus. He can help you process the aches and emotions. Instead of absorbing the hurt and letting it spill out on other people, you can pour out your heart to him.

Financial Feasibility

This journey takes a significant financial toll as well. Even without fertility treatments, the expenses add up from buying pregnancy tests in bulk. Here's a quick rundown of potential costs in the United States:

- One cycle of IVF on average costs about $20,000.[2] Additional clinic baseline fees can be up to $10,000.[3]
- Adoption can cost anywhere from $5,000 (for fostering to adopt, depending on where you live) to $50,000 (international).[4]
- Domestic adoption costs $43,000 on average.[5]
- Embryo adoption costs are variable, with a range of $2,500 to $6,000 for the frozen embryo transfer (not including medications) and $2,000 to $3,500 for the adoption home study fees.[6]

You must first consider whether you have the money for the path you're pursuing. Perhaps you've had to work extra hours or jobs, or you and your husband are both more stressed from the burden of providing. These realities can interfere with our time, energy, and care for our spouse and ourselves.

During one IUI, I had overstimulated, and the fertility clinic told us we could start IVF the following day. However, financially it was not feasible for us. We knew our line in the sand, and we weren't willing to exert our wants over the cost. God gives provision for his will. Although we could have called every friend and family member and tried to make it happen, we knew that wasn't the best.

In his parable of the talents in Matthew 25:14–30, Jesus described believers as stewards, meaning overseers of his possessions and affairs. So we must ask ourselves, are we using what God has given us faithfully, for his sake? That's not an easy question, but it's important since fertility treatments, adoption, and the expenses to continue this journey for an extended time require a substantial financial investment.

If you are feeling the burden, know that God can bring peace in this matter. Seek wise counsel, participate in a Financial Peace University course,[7] and take smart steps together. Then give yourself grace, knowing the Lord leads you.

Relational Toll

In our single-focused vision, we can't see ourselves correctly, let alone those around us. As a result, we struggle to receive or extend grace to ourselves and others.

As discussed in chapter 24, if we are hypersensitive to the extent that we think others are trying to hurt us, then we will likely be unable to forgive them for their carelessness. Perhaps you are at a point where you need a break or need to take a step back to reevaluate the toll your journey is having on your relationships.

As believers, we need to consider our witness. In Romans 14 and 15, Paul urged us not to become a stumbling block to others. Be aware that your life will be a living testimony for God through the decisions you make about resolving your infertility.

We also need to take into account the witness of our marriages. Through our marriage relationships, we display Christ's love and the church to those around us. This topic has been the heaviest in my heart within our ministry. I am brokenhearted to watch too many marriages suffer when they don't have to. Many spouses forget to put their marriage before their attempts to have a baby. But marriage came first. I know that for many of us, this is not the order we tend to fall into during our infertility journeys. We need to guard against letting the goal of having a baby hijack our marital relationships.

Spiritual Reckoning

Is the pursuit of God our priority? As followers of Jesus Christ, our lives should display our hearts. Where our hearts are, our lives will follow.

We must take account spiritually of the actions and choices we make on this journey before a holy God. We must consider whether our steps are acceptable and beneficial in God's sight. In 1 Corinthians 6:12, Paul said, "'Everything is permissible for me,' but not everything is beneficial" (csb). God's wisdom and guidance should be what we seek above others' advice.

While imprisoned and near his death, Paul wrote to the believers in Philippi, rejoicing and encouraging them that knowing Christ must be their ultimate goal. He said, "I count everything as loss compared to the priceless privilege and supreme advantage of knowing Christ Jesus my Lord [and of growing more deeply and thoroughly acquainted with Him—a joy unequaled]. For His sake I have lost everything . . . so that I may gain Christ, and may be found in Him [believing and relying on Him]" (Philippians 3:8–9 AMP).

Are you living for Christ? Is knowing him personally the goal of your life? If not, then he is second at best. Ask yourself, am I investing more time, prayers, effort, and heart into the pursuit of parenthood than into my relationship with my heavenly Father?

Counting the Cost

This chapter has been more direct in nature. I probably have seemed less friendly, but only because I am the friend who must tell you what you need to know before you go too far.

I care about you too much to let you fall because of this season of infertility. If it's too heavy a burden to carry, then turn and trust Jesus. He calls us to come to him if we are weary, for his burden is light and we can find rest in his grace (Matthew 11:28–30).

I know you want a child, and that is a good, beautiful desire. But to what extent are you willing to go? Is pursuing a baby coming at the detriment of yourself, your marriage, and your life now and in the future?

If you feel stuck, unsure, angry with God, or are asking God all the "why?" questions, then it may be the time to pause, take a breath, and rest. I did this several times in our journey, not because it made sense but because I had to tend to my soul. Choose to take care of yourself and those around you. Following Philippians 3:8 is not easy. But honestly, there is nothing more important (or surpassing in worth) in all of life than knowing (and being known) by Christ Jesus, *your* Lord.

Reflect

- Do you recognize the woman in the mirror? Have you been treating your body in a God-honoring manner? Take a moment to assess your pain level, physically and emotionally.

_____

_____

_____

_____

_____

- Does your current path fit in your budget? Have you or your spouse had to work extra hours or jobs to make ends meet? Describe any stress brought on by the financial burden of infertility.

_____

_____

_____

_____

_____

- Are the actions you're taking God-honoring? Are they moving you toward deeper connection with the Lord, or pushing you away from him? Ask him to search your heart and reveal anything that needs to be realigned toward him.

_____

_____

_____

_____

_____

Pray

Dear Jesus, I'm tired of carrying all the burdens of this journey. Infertility has taken so much from me that I can't recognize myself anymore. I'm not sure if the wait is still worth it. Please help me examine the costs and make wise decisions. Give me courage to believe that pursuing a baby is good, but it's not as important as the privilege of pursuing you, my Savior and Friend. Thank you for taking up the cross to free me from the burden on my soul. I want to seek you from this step forward, wherever you lead.

Act

Identify which area has taken the biggest toll: physical (your body), spiritual (your relationship with Jesus), or relational (your spouse and/or other friends and family). Then put a plan in place to take one step in a better direction today. Remember, you just asked God to help you carry this and lead you—he will!

28

Two Pink Lines

Come and see what God has done, his
awesome deeds for mankind!

Psalm 66:5

Trigger warning: Read this chapter when you're ready or able.

If we'd had any inclination or feeling that I (Kelley) was pregnant, we would have taken the test together. But I ended up texting my husband instead: "I know you don't want to be told this way but . . ." I attached a photo of the positive pregnancy test.

He quickly responded, "What?" and then called: "Wait, seriously? Call the clinic and go in to make sure!"

The office was surprised too, saying to come right in and get blood drawn. By early afternoon they called to confirm that I was, indeed, pregnant!

I was in total disbelief. After all the tears shed and resources poured into our infertility, I felt the need to pinch myself to believe the two pink lines that I had longed to see so many times.

If and when the test comes up positive, it's as though we don't know how to accept that it finally happened after all this time. Or maybe it feels too good to be true after so many months of pain. So we don't allow ourselves to fully believe or celebrate it. Instead, we put up a guard just in case something were to happen. After waiting so long or experiencing a miscarriage, it's easy for us to question: "Is this real?" "How could I be pregnant?"

On the heels of pregnancy shock comes fear. After my pregnancy was confirmed, the following weeks were land mines of fear as each new symptom sparked a concern and a call to the doctor's nurse. Even the *lack of* symptoms taunted me that I was losing my baby. I wanted to believe and be joyful, but I was cautious after only a few weeks and felt like a seesaw of praise and doubt.

Meanwhile, a still, small voice echoed in my heart Jeremiah 32:27: "I am the LORD, the God of all mankind. Is anything too hard for me?"

Fight for Joy and Against Fear

Experiencing pregnancy after infertility brings a wave of conflicting feelings to an already emotionally intense process. We attempt to quickly put aside our waiting and grief for a joyous new season. But, inevitably, it's a struggle to switch gears from grieving to celebrating. That's the difficulty we find ourselves in.

Joy is not an easy emotion. The only way to have joy is to fight for it. Even if you become pregnant, you may think those two pink lines will be the answer that makes your joy overflow, yet that's not necessarily the case. Instead, I found that my heart was still in need of healing as I wrestled with many different emotions.

Once pregnant, I struggled with the complicated emotion of fear. There are many things we can be fearful of during pregnancy: losing the baby, having pregnancy complications, birthing issues, congenital disabilities, eating the right things, uncertainty about what's ahead, and not knowing how to raise a child.

Fear is tricky, like a weed that hides and tries to choke out a flowering plant. I found that even deeper than my fear of losing the baby was my fear of being out of control and not able to know the next step of the plan. It's difficult to enjoy pregnancy if we assume every symptom is bad and every lack of symptom is catastrophic.

Pregnancy itself can make you bonkers from all the dos and don'ts, and you can easily slip back into grasping for control. There are reasonable measures your doctor may suggest, and in which you should follow their wisdom. But most importantly, choose to trust God each day and give every fear to him. He is the one who holds life together.

As we learned in chapter 2, fighting fear requires us to "take captive every thought to make it obedient to Christ" (2 Corinthians 10:5). The Message version renders this verse as "fitting every loose thought and emotion and impulse into the structure of life shaped by Christ."

Ultimately, I discovered that when the object of my joy was simply the thing I was desiring (to be pregnant), I was left on the battlefield of all these emotions. But when I took my thoughts captive and focused on the true source of my joy (Jesus, how he had carried me through this painful season of waiting, how he was the one who had blessed me with new life), then I could truly celebrate.

It's easier to have joy when we aren't tossed around by every thought or concern but instead are held steady by Jesus Christ (Ephesians 4:14). Psalm 33 is our hope for you in this new season. This psalm starts by reminding us to sing joyfully, praise God, and shout for joy because he is faithful in all he does. It ends with the realization that our hearts can rejoice in him, for we trust in his holy name.

Learn How to Celebrate

I wanted to enjoy every day of this pregnancy—unlike the last pregnancy, which I never enjoyed fully because I thought I was being smart in protecting myself.

Celebrating all God has done and bringing him glory can become part of the healing process that God is working in your heart and soul. Paul commanded us in Romans 12:15 to "rejoice with those who rejoice" and "mourn with those who mourn." You're now on the rejoicing side. No matter how you got pregnant, this new life is a miracle from God!

Solomon declared that everything under heaven has a season, a time, and a purpose in his ways (Ecclesiastes 3:1–8). If you have seen two pink lines, then this is the time to celebrate the wonder of what only God can do. It's good, right, and God-honoring to be excited about this new little life that he has knit together in your womb. So let praises lift, worship him, and overflow with joy about what our God has done.

I know it will be hard thinking about when, where, and how you will share your good news. And though you shouldn't be afraid to share your news, remember how it made you feel to find out about others' announcements. There are ways to share and not forget the wisdom, empathy, and sensitivity you gained during infertility. Let your moment of celebrating by sharing help others see Christ's goodness from what you've been through and how hard it was for you.

I've seen beautiful community in our Waiting in Hope support groups as women become pregnant and the group rallies around them to rejoice and praise. We encourage our leaders to facilitate an atmosphere of vulnerability and encouragement, a safe space to learn to support one another and celebrate.

Pregnancy after infertility does not immediately remove the struggle to get there. We still need others to walk beside us and hold us up if needed. So stay connected in a community that will be there for you, even when pregnant. It's powerful when together we learn to rejoice and have hope in God's wonders.

Mourning to Dancing

In the Lord's provision and loving-kindness, as I was writing this chapter, my sister-in-law texted that she had just had her blood drawn and would know the outcome of her last IVF cycle that afternoon. Later, while still writing, I answered her call to hear, "I'm pregnant!"

I found myself squealing and crying with pure relief, excitement, and joy! Thank you, Lord! Her journey has been grueling, full of medical issues and roadblocks. But, as Matthew 19:26 says, "With man this is impossible, but with God all things are possible." So this news was entirely God's mighty hand at work.

God has given me a new perspective after my journey with infertility. I've realized that I truly had no control over getting pregnant. Instead, it was ultimately God's hand working. As a result, I no longer claimed ownership or felt like this baby was mine to lose, which helped me truly trust and be confident in the blessing of all God was doing.

"You have turned for me my mourning into dancing; you have loosed my sackcloth and clothed me with gladness, that my glory may sing your praise and not be silent. O LORD my God, I will give thanks to you forever!" (Psalm 30:11–12 ESV).

Reflect

- If God has done a mighty work and you are pregnant, do you feel able to celebrate, or are you cautious, fearful, or feeling guilty comparing your situation to those of infertility sisters?

_____

_____

_____

_____

- Can you relate to any of the fears listed? Write down your specific worries.

_____

_____

_____

_____

_____

- Fighting fear requires us to "take captive every thought to make it obedient to Christ" (2 Corinthians 10:5). What thoughts, emotions, or impulses do you need to take captive and surrender to Christ's authority?

_____

_____

_____

_____

_____

Pray

Lord, thank you! You are so great and worthy of all my praise. You created life in me from nothing and you have the power and the authority to sustain it. I pray that you will put your hand over this life, this baby you have given me, and keep him or her growing. Thank you, Father! I praise you for your mighty hand that saves, rescues, redeems, and has always loved me. Help me trust you with this life and enjoy every moment of this baby we've been given. May we trust you with our hearts for your protection of our pregnancy.

Act

If you are pregnant, talk to your husband and together ask God to help you announce your pregnancy with joy and sensitivity. Make a plan for when and how you'll share your news. Here's an example:

- Tell your closest loved ones.
- Tell your friends and family who are still in the trenches of infertility and miscarriage. Think about whether it's best to call, send an email, or tell them in person. (Consider whether texting might catch them off-guard.)
- Optional: Make an announcement on social media. We encourage you to consider sharing about the hard journey you've traveled to get here. God can use your story to bring him glory and encourage others.

29

Born in Your Heart

See, I am doing a new thing! Now it springs up;
do you not perceive it? I am making a way in the
wilderness and streams in the wasteland.

Isaiah 43:19

I (Jenn) will never forget how one mom at an adoption conference described her journey to parenthood. An audience member asked how she felt about waiting longer to adopt compared to her friends who got pregnant easily. She shrugged and replied, "They took a flight. We went by boat."

Her answer offered a helpful way to think about how I could become a mom. God had given me the desire for adoption before I got married. My plan was to have biological children, then adopt children. To use the analogy, I thought I'd take a plane first, then book a boat trip. But God had a different itinerary.

I know adoption is a sensitive topic. I'm sure you're tired of hearing family members, friends, pastors, or even doctors tell you, "Just adopt." Maybe your story is similar to my friend Kim's. Before infertility, she'd never thought about adoption because she always expected to have biological children. "I was completely blindsided, and I stayed in shock and denial for years," Kim said. "God had to soften my heart to adoption."

However you feel about adoption, it probably wasn't your plan A. But with this unexpected turn in your journey, God is giving you another opportunity to trust him. Proverbs 16:9 says, "The heart of man plans his way, but the LORD establishes his steps" (ESV). Your plans might be unraveling, but God's plan A won't fail. Infertility could be his way of redirecting your steps toward adoption.

While adoption also holds unknowns and potential heartbreak, I encourage you to examine this path. God can use adoption to grow families in creative, redemptive ways even with the complexities involved.

The word *adoption* is used in reference to several family-growing options, including foster care, foster-to-adopt, and embryo adoption. Each option involves ethical, emotional, and relational issues beyond what we can address in one chapter. For our purposes, we'll focus on the process of welcoming a child through domestic adoption and international adoption.

Five Questions to Guide Your Decision

As you consider adoption, the maze of information can be overwhelming. To help you think about the decision, let's look at five questions to talk through with your spouse.

Are You and Your Husband on the Same Page?

Adoption can bring out strong feelings from both spouses. For example, a wife might be ready to jump into the adoption process, while her husband is reluctant or rejects the idea—and these roles can be reversed. I've seen times when the husband wanted to adopt, but the wife was opposed.

Marital disagreements over adoption are gut-wrenching. Ask the Lord to help you be patient and hear what your husband has to say. Keep in mind you're both carrying individual hopes and fears, along with your own pre-conceptions about adoption.

Being on the same page *doesn't* mean the two of you must agree completely or immediately. Instead, you reach the same page by going over pros and cons together, talking about your desires together, reviewing other options together, and praying for wisdom together. The point is to move toward a decision *together* with humility and love.

Have You Processed Your Infertility Grief?

Many adoption agencies require couples to sign a document saying they've dealt with the grief of not having biological children. The purpose is to make sure they're emotionally prepared to move forward with adopting a child.

It's wise to address the emotional trauma of infertility and miscarriage, regardless of what you decide about adoption. See a licensed professional counselor or therapist familiar with infertility, talk with a pastor or trusted friend, and practice positive coping skills.

Like all grief, infertility grief isn't an obstacle you "get over." Instead, you look at the emotions, sort through them, and make your heart tender toward what God has in store for you.

My friend Kim spent eight hours one day weeping on her couch. Although she continued to release her emotions after that day, she stopped living in denial. "You slowly gain momentum to become a parent, and that desire is greater than your desire to be pregnant and birth a child with your own body," she said.

Do You See Adoption as Second-Best to Having "Your Own Child"?

Think of the analogy we talked about at the beginning of the chapter. Just as a boat isn't a worse way to travel than a plane, neither is adoption inferior to getting pregnant. Both pregnancy and adoption are good, God-ordained ways to grow your family.

You don't need to feel ashamed for wanting a biological child. But take a moment to imagine you were adopted. How would you feel about the phrase "your own child"? An adopted child isn't a consolation prize for the biological child you wanted. All children are created by God and worthy of love, dignity, and care. When you adopt a child, you make a declaration of belonging. You're his or her parent. He or she is *your own child* brought to life through another woman's womb.

Hear this vital distinction: adoption fulfills the desire to be a parent, but it doesn't fulfill the desire for a child who carries your genes. If you're wrestling with the thought of never getting pregnant or having a biological child, you might have more grieving to do before pursuing adoption. Adopted children deserve parents who desire them for the precious humans they are.

Have You Weighed the Investment?

Adoption is a long-haul commitment. People tend to focus on the financial cost of adoption, which, granted, can add up to thousands of dollars.

But the emotional investment doesn't always get addressed when couples consider adoption. For all the emotions you've poured out over infertility, you'll have more feelings to process over adoption. With adoption, you take on the responsibility to help your adopted child work through their own complex emotions. Your child will have layers of identity and relational issues to unwrap over time—maybe a whole lifetime. If you pursue transracial and/or international adoption, that adds layers of grief, trauma, and cultural influences.

It can be intimidating when you think of the sum of the emotional investment of adoption. But remember the burdens of adoption aren't yours to bear alone. Jesus has walked with you through infertility. He'll keep walking with you through adoption. So cast these complicated cares on him (1 Peter 5:7). Nothing is beyond his power to overcome.

Do You Want to Adopt?

You need to ask yourself and your husband whether you really want to adopt. Let these three truths help guide your response:

- Adoption is a grace-filled path to becoming a parent.
- Adoption isn't for everyone.
- Adoption is a calling from the Lord.

The Bible tells all Christians to care for orphans (including functional orphans who need loving, stable homes). James 1:27 says, "Religion that God our Father accepts as pure and faultless is this: to look after orphans and widows in their distress and to keep oneself from being polluted by the world." Orphan care can happen in many ways—donating to charities, volunteering, and supporting foster families, just to name a few. The Bible doesn't tell all Christians or all infertile Christians they must adopt.

Adoption isn't your obligation because you're struggling with infertility. Not only is this view incorrect, but it isn't a good mindset to carry into the process of adding a child to your family through adoption. God can and does change our desires. Pray and seek his wisdom, then wait and see if he leads you in this direction.

A Worthy Path

Neither adoption nor pregnancy can cure the wounds of infertility. You need Jesus to heal the losses of your vision of motherhood. The beauty of adoption is that it cures your childlessness and so much more. For the adoptive parents, the adopted child, and potentially the birth family, God moves through loss to multiply love.

I'll say this from personal experience: adoption is 100 percent worth every tear you shed over your aching womb. Ask the Lord if this is a new desire he wants to plant in your heart.

Reflect

- What have you done to address your infertility grief? Do the hard work of naming the dreams you're grieving.

_____

_____

_____

_____

_____

- What may be causing you to consider adoption? Are you out of medical options? Are you feeling drawn toward vulnerable children? Your answers don't have to be mutually exclusive. It's important to examine the "whys" of your process.

_____

_____

_____

_____

_____

- What aspects of adoption scare you? What makes you excited? Your answers could provide insight into how God might be shifting your desires.

_____

_____

_____

_____

_____

Pray

Dear Lord, I know you're Father to the fatherless (Psalm 68:5). I praise you for wrapping your arms of protection around vulnerable children. As my heavenly Father, you've seen me wrestle with the changes to my family plans. I'm not sure yet if you're leading us to adoption. This path has so many issues to work through, I admit it feels overwhelming. Give me faith to follow your lead. Help me do the necessary research and, through the Spirit's wisdom, assess if this is a path that's right for us. Thank you for loving me as your own child.

Act

Have you and your husband talked about any of the five questions in this chapter? Spend some time discussing each one.

Search for stories from the perspectives of different people involved in adoption: an adoptive parent, an adoptee, a birth mother, and an adoption professional. If you don't know anyone, search the Waiting in Hope blog (waitinginhopeinfertility.com/blog) for adoption posts.

30

Different Can Be Beautiful

I have come that they may have life, and have it to the full.

John 10:10

If you haven't watched the Disney Pixar movie *Up*, consider yourself warned: you'll need a box of tissues to get through the opening scene.

Up starts with a montage showing how childhood friends Carl and Ellie fall in love and get married. Their romance unfolds like a fairy tale until Ellie gets pregnant and loses the baby. The couple grows old together without any children in the picture. Then Ellie passes away, leaving Carl to sit alone in his armchair. The crotchety widower eventually comes to terms with his grief, but not before reaching a breaking point. Overwhelmed by the challenges life has thrown at him, Carl yells, "I didn't ask for any of this!"[1]

Doesn't that echo the anguish of infertility? "I didn't ask to be barren!" No one dreams of struggling to get pregnant. Our version of a beautiful life is a life that goes according to our plans.

Dear one, I (Jenn) am sure you're aware that life isn't a fairy tale. Maybe you've hit what feels like your last dead end in the adoption process. Or your husband told you he couldn't handle trying anymore. Or perhaps you're single, waiting to see if God will write marriage or motherhood into your story. Whatever your situation, you might be considering the path of childlessness.

Though the decision involves grief, you can remain childless and still flourish.[2] Think of what Jesus told his disciples: "I am the vine; you are the branches. If you remain in me and I in you, you will bear much fruit; apart from me you can do nothing" (John 15:5). The key to thriving is staying connected to the Vine. Every woman who loves Jesus can live a meaningful, abundant life—even if it's not the life she planned.

Stories of Unexpected Goodness

Childlessness brings opportunities you wouldn't have otherwise. If God is leading you on this path, he'll show you new and vibrant ways to experience his goodness. While all journeys are different, it can be helpful to have examples of what childlessness can look like. I want to share with you stories from three women who tell how God filled them with love overflowing.

Anna's Story

Going through an unsuccessful IVF cycle not only crushed Anna's hopes, but it also almost cost Anna her life. The forty-two-year-old and her husband tried another frozen transfer that didn't result in implantation. Doctors eventually advised them to stop all fertility treatments due to her continuing complications. After an adoption possibility fell through, the couple recognized the need to slow down and grieve.

During their break, Anna realized God was leading her to enroll in graduate school and start new roles as a therapist and ministry leader. Her decision came through a process of seeking wise counsel and crying out to the Lord.

"When everything was seemingly slammed, with locked doors and shattered dreams, I sobbed one night, 'I don't know what you're doing, or why all of this is happening. But please, whatever you do, don't waste my hurt,'" Anna said. "The parenting door has remained firmly shut, but so many other doors have opened. I just keep saying, 'Okay, I guess this is where we're going next!' and stepping through."

Anna put in her graduate work and earned a master's degree in marriage and family therapy. She recently started her own private practice in California. God also prompted her to create a safe space at her church where people could share their infertility stories.

A supportive community helped Anna accept this new path. For her, coming to terms with childlessness involved accepting the grief. "It's okay to be sad about all of the losses I experienced and wonder who those babies would have been and who I might have been as a parent," she said. "Jesus was sad when things were sad, and he showed the value of seeking comfort and also lamenting and weeping during sad and difficult times."

Nicolet's Story

Loss and shame weighed on Nicolet long before she faced infertility. Raised in a violent environment, she became an emancipated minor at age fifteen and, at twenty-four, had an unplanned pregnancy that ended in abortion. Years later Nicolet spiraled into depression when she and her husband began struggling to conceive and build their family. It wasn't until she joined a post-abortion care support group that she truly believed Jesus had washed her clean and would redeem her pain—past and present. "To combat the shame, hopelessness, isolation, despair, and deep sorrow, I held on to his promise of beauty for ashes," she said.

Nicolet, who's now forty-seven, committed to trust the Lord throughout her waiting journey, even after an IVF cycle produced only one viable egg and the resulting embryo didn't reach the blastocyst stage for transfer. She considered embryo adoption and egg donation, but God led her to surrender her plans. Now instead of expecting him to deliver answers, she's learning to accept and share his love.

As Nicolet has worked through her difficult past, her heart has been drawn toward children who come from broken homes. When her church started a program for mentoring foster youth, Nicolet jumped in immediately. She was matched with two at-risk teenagers in 2017 and 2019, and has continued to meet with them when they ask to see her. Through these relationships, God has shown Nicolet how she can help break cycles of generational trauma and be a mother in a different way. "Jesus is guiding me to question, 'Are you okay if they never call you mom? Can you be who you are for your mentees and vulnerable children?'" she said. "And I'm getting to the place where that's enough."

Dana's Story

Surrendering to God didn't come easily for Dana. She and her husband decided to stop fertility treatments after exploring all viable medical options without success. However, daily prayer, meetings with her spiritual director, and the support of friends within the Waiting in Hope online support group have helped forty-five-year-old Dana grow to trust God more fully with her journey. "I'm a control freak and plan everything to a T," she said. "Realizing this was something I could not plan was a pivotal change in my faith."

Dana also learned the truth about how God sees her. Early in her journey, she felt like God was punishing her for not trying to conceive a child when she was younger. Her feelings of grief, anxiety, and shame took time to process. But it was worth the effort to grasp that the Lord loves her and was walking with her through the most challenging season of her life up to then.

Dana has witnessed God's glory and grace in sharing her story on social media. "I was able to touch other women going through similar journeys and connect with friends who had an infertility story, and I didn't even know about it," Dana said. "God used my story and pain to give others strength and courage. It's been so life-giving to experience those moments. And now I can share that being husband and wife makes us a family. A life without children is still a life, and I do what I can to uplift others so they see what a beautiful life it can be."

Adventure Ahead

Toward the end of *Up*, Carl finds a note from his beloved wife: "Thanks for the adventure. Now go have a new one! Love, Ellie." Carl's unplanned adventure leads him to a young boy in need of a friend, mentor, and father figure. As they journey together, Carl learns how to honor the past while embracing the relationships in front of him.[3]

This sweet movie offers a picture of God's invitation as you consider the path of childlessness: *Come, let's go on an adventure. It doesn't match your plans, which I know is hard to accept. You can't see what lies ahead. But remember, I'm going with you. If you trust me, I'll guide you to the tops of my beauty. Just take my hand, and I'll lead you on an adventure called faith.*

Reflect

- Are you wondering if you're near the end of your wait? It's better to confront your fears head-on than to stuff them inside.

_____

_____

_____

_____

_____

- What areas of life do you wish you could control? Name the things you're holding on to, then pray and ask God to help you loosen your grip.

_____

_____

_____

_____

_____

- Author and speaker Jill Briscoe said, "Your mission field is the area between your own two feet at any given time."4 How are you serving God right now? Think about where he placed you and ways you can share your faith there. Turning your focus to the opportunities in front of you can help you resist worries about the what-ifs of considering childlessness.

_____

_____

_____

_____

_____

Pray

Dear Jesus, I praise you for being my Savior, Redeemer, and Friend. I know that you see me grieving the life I thought I'd have by now. As I think about the path of childlessness, please give me wisdom and courage. Help me believe that I can still enjoy your abundance even if I don't have children. Keep my heart close to yours so I can share the joy of being reborn. I want to trust that you'll make my life beautiful, in your own time and your own ways.

Act

Where is the Lord calling you to take an adventure? Take a leap and dream with God. Look at a map or globe and find a city or region you'd love to explore someday. As you look up information about the place you chose, think of how God created the marvelous sights there. This will give you an exercise in imagination, picturing the excitement of following God wherever he leads.

31

How to Wait in Hope

We wait in hope for the LORD; he is our help and our shield. In him our hearts rejoice, for we trust in his holy name. May your unfailing love be with us, LORD, even as we put our hope in you.

Psalm 33:20–22

Well done, friend. You've reached the end of our journey together. We know it wasn't easy—because nothing about infertility is easy.

Look at all the ground we covered in this book: the emotions, spiritual issues, relationships, and paths to resolve infertility. This is why we call waiting a journey. Rather than sink into despair, you put one foot in front of the other, pressing through the hard things in a hopeful direction.

However long it takes, your journey of waiting *will* end. You can't see the other side yet. It might feel like you'll never get there. We struggled with those feelings too. Thankfully, our feelings don't change God's good plan for us.

Both of us have walked this road ourselves and alongside others. We've had the honor of watching God do amazing work in women's journeys:

- He performed miracles in empty wombs, broken marriages, and wandering hearts.

- He filled some women's arms with biological babies and some with adopted babies or older children.
- He led women to mentor foster youth, serve on mission trips, support refugees, and rescue girls from trafficking.

In our years of infertility ministry, we have discovered something true about waiting. To make the most of your journey, you learn lessons along the way.

Infertility is a training season. It's not downtime or wasted time. God is working all things for your good *now* (Romans 8:28). The tools he's providing can help you live with purpose in this season and beyond.

One of our favorite authors, Elisabeth Elliot, wrote this about the loss of her first husband, missionary Jim Elliot: "Suffering is an irreplaceable medium through which I learned an indispensable truth."[1]

Waiting *is* suffering. Suffering brings pain and also reveals truth. God shines truth through the broken pieces of our journeys. Before we finish this time together, we want to share three lessons we learned from women who let the wait shape them.

You Can Trust God

"I've had the hardest time with trusting. I just didn't trust that God was still good (to me)," said Hannah, who leads a Waiting in Hope support group in her community. Infertility brings you here, where the rubber of your faith meets the road.

Waiting in hope is about *choosing* to trust God. Either he is who he says he is, or he isn't. Either he is trustworthy, or he isn't.

I (Kelley) spent months fighting for my faith. Today I can say with full confidence that God is more than trustworthy. He chose us when we didn't deserve it (Ephesians 1:4) and he gives us every ounce of the strength we need to trust him (Psalm 28:7). By his goodness, he helps our broken hearts see through his eyes. By his faithfulness, he matures our faith. He disciples us through our waiting just as Jesus discipled the men who traveled with him. No longer do we simply *know about* the Messiah; now we *know* him and walk hand in hand with our Shepherd.

We pick up lessons from waiting and then apply them to the next journey. I continually return to the renewed faith gained in my years of infertility training. The same whispers from God ask me, *Do you trust me, Kelley?* And I say, "Yes. I choose you, Lord."

You Can Use Your Pain

Knowing you're not alone makes a difference in your wait. When infertility knocks you down, you need someone to lift your eyes to the Rock. That's part of our mission at Waiting in Hope. We want to help you get into a community of encouragement.

I (Jenn) can name specific people God placed in my life to keep me tethered to hope. Their support carried me through the worst drops of the emotional roller coaster. Later, when I wasn't as lost in my grief, I saw these people from another angle. They were fellow sufferers, offering me comfort through their wounds.

This is how God flips the script on pain. The heartbreak he allows in our lives molds us into messengers of hope. Your pain isn't about you. I know that's tough to hear. But the sooner you realize this purpose for your wait, the more wonders you'll see.

Transformation happens when you allow God to turn your struggle into passion for his kingdom. The Spirit who raised Jesus from the grave can resurrect your ash heap of dreams to spread his glory and save lives. Isn't it surprising and wonderful that God works through us weak and needy daughters? I pray you'll experience more of his grace as you use your pain and show others they're not alone.

You Can Find Hope

The "what" of your wait matters. You're not waiting for a new car, a raise at work, or the latest season of your favorite Netflix show. You're waiting for a little person who calls you "mama." A child is worth the days, months, years, and sob sessions of your wait. We join you in praying and asking the Lord to bring new life into the world and into your home.

With God, there's always a deeper layer to our circumstances. It's true that a baby can give you joy, love, a full-time commitment, and a picture of God's goodness. What a baby can't give you is hope.

Only Jesus gives true hope. Hope that pierces darkness. Hope that heals. Hope that fills your utmost longings.

Paul shared his hope in Philippians 4:11–13: "I am not saying this because I am in need, for I have learned to be content whatever the circumstances. I know what it is to be in need, and I know what it is to have plenty. I have learned the secret of being content in any and every situation, whether well fed or hungry, whether living in plenty or in want. I can do all this through him who gives me strength."

Paul's source of strength and his source of contentment were one and the same, found in Christ alone. Notice God didn't shout a command to Paul: "Just be content!" Instead, Paul said he had to *learn* the secret of being content. Contentment came to him gradually. It was a *secret* that took time to understand.

Infertility is your season for learning how to be content. You can ache for a child and still be full. I (Kelley) have seen women come alive even within the desolation of waiting. They became lighter, more fully themselves as they drew closer to Jesus. One friend of mine shared that she didn't want her waiting to end. Infertility was the holy ground where she experienced the nearness of her Savior.

Our greatest hope is that you'll see Jesus in your wait. He will give you the courage to proclaim, "It is well," even when you're not well. Like Shadrach, Meshach, and Abednego in Daniel 3, we can say, "We know our God can, but *even if he does not,* he is still good. And *even then* we will only praise our Lord God (emphasis added)."

You Have a Choice

We don't get to choose our journeys. But we do get to choose how we wait. Will your wait be aimless, with you grasping for things you can't actually control? Or will you find purpose in the One who saved you and sustains your life?

Choosing to wait in hope with the Lord may sound lofty, but it's not. You can, because the Holy Spirit will empower you. Your job is to ask and accept. "Lord, help me. I want to choose you and do this with you, not by myself."

Choose to slow down, look at your heavenly Father, and believe that he cares. Then choose to grip his hand tightly and walk with him through this hard now.

He will carry you with hope that lasts forever.

Reflect

- How have you seen God move in your wait? Spend time celebrating what the Lord has done through this journey.

_____

_____

_____

_____

_____

- If we had to pick three words for you to take away from this book (besides _waiting in hope_), they'd be _seek_, _trust_, and _share_. Which words would you choose?

_____

_____

_____

_____

_____

- How can you wait in hope today?

_____

_____

_____

_____

_____

Pray

Lord Jesus, you're my hope. I thank you for dying to rescue me from trying to live for myself and through my own strength. You've given me the joy of your presence in my waiting. I see now how your unfailing love is with me, even as I continue this long, hard journey. Grow my faith to ask, seek, and trust you with what you have planned for my life. Make my wait be about you.

Act

Go back and read a few of your Reflect notes from each of the four sections of the book. See how your heart has progressed from beginning to end. Then thank God for all he's doing in your life.

Acknowledgments

This book is the fruit of God's work through our waiting. Lord Jesus, you made a way when we couldn't see any possible way forward. We give you all the glory for inspiring, motivating, and sustaining us to share your message of hope.

To the team at W Publishing, thank you for seeing the need for a Christian book on infertility. You invested in two first-time authors and enabled us to reach a wider audience than we imagined. Kyle, if we're honest, we didn't expect to work with a male acquisitions editor. Yet God knew what he was doing, giving us a wise guide through the publishing process. Thank you for committing to serve our community.

Blythe, you took us under your wing and led us into a new, intimidating world. Thank you for being our advocate and partnering in this labor of love. And thanks to Sarah for pioneering our path to publishing by connecting us with Blythe.

We couldn't have written this book without our Waiting in Hope Ministries team. L-swag (Laura), our master task juggler, thank you for handling details for the book while continuing to run the ministry. We also owe shout-outs to Justin, Hallie, and Jaclyn for helping write the invaluable appendices. This book came to life through the encouragement, counsel, and prayer support of our advisory team. Special thanks to our research assistants, Stephanie and Kelly O., who dug for answers to our burning questions.

To the women we interviewed, thank you for making this book what it is—a collection of voices speaking hope to the brokenhearted. What a privilege you gave us to share your stories.

Both of us leaned on our families and friends while fulfilling this calling. Thank you for your prayers, texts, and teletherapy sessions. We needed you to remind us why our work matters.

Justin, thank you for believing in this book, so much so that the Lord revealed to you years ago that a book would happen, even though I (Kelley) laughed in disbelief. I'm blessed by so many of my dearest cheering me on, believing in this calling, praying over this work, and declaring it was needed and we had to write it. Becky, thank you for not letting me give up and for reminding me I am a writer of what God has written in my heart. Carter and Greyson, I've been blessed by your loving and encouraging support, for giving me time and space while repeatedly asking, "Is your book done yet?" Boys, I'm happy to say it's finally done! I've loved showing you that obedience to God's call is often unexpected, but he does the work through us.

Colin, if it were up to me (Jenn), I would have listed you as third coauthor. You pushed me, consoled me, kept me supplied with dairy-free ice cream, and believed in me when I wanted to quit. I thank God for you and the gift of being your wife. Calvin, Linus, and Harry, you crazy boys made writing a book more complicated, but also lifted my spirits. I pray you'll know the love of Jesus and how he writes the best stories. I'm also grateful for the people God placed in my life to help make this book a reality: my soul sister Rebekah and Writing with Grace friends, who spurred me on in faith; Em, who nannied my unpredictable baby; and Bonnie, who opened her home so I could have a quiet place to hear my own thoughts.

For every person who supported us in our infertility and book journeys, thank you for carrying us to the finish line. We're still in shock that we got to do this—only by God's grace and the love of his people.

About the Authors

Kelley Ramsey is the founder and visionary of Waiting in Hope Ministries. She is a speaker and leader with a heart for seeing women come to love and live for the Lord more intimately. Kelley and her husband, Justin, and their two sons live in The Woodlands, Texas. When they're not hosting friends or traveling, you'll find them at their happy place on the lake. They're looking forward to their next big adventure as a waiting adoptive family. Follow her @kelramsey on Facebook and Instagram.

Jenn Hesse is the content director of Waiting in Hope Ministries. She leads local Bible studies and has a passion for shepherding hurting women. Jenn and her husband, Colin, and their three sons live in the lush Willamette Valley, Oregon, where they enjoy swimming, exploring parks, and racking up late fees at the library. Find her at jennhesse.com and @jennmhesse on Facebook, Twitter, and Instagram.

APPENDIX A

For Waiting Husbands

by Justin Ramsey

As a man, the idea of not being able to have kids and become a father was never on my radar. In fact, it was the opposite for many years after Kelley and I got married. I was trying hard to *not* have kids until I thought we "were ready," and I had all my ducks lined up.

However, as we started trying to become pregnant with no success, this came as a big kick in the gut to the planner side of me. Months passed, then years, with fertility specialists, surgeries, treatments, multiple miscarriages, and lots of sadness, frustration, and anger along the way. For years we felt isolated and alone. We were jealous of our friends who had no trouble getting pregnant. It was a dark time for me, mostly because I was in hiding.

But what was I to do? That's just it. This wasn't about me or something I could do. You can't "fix" infertility. This is extremely hard to accept as a man. We want to fix and make things better for those we love. Yet I couldn't fix our situation or my wife's roller coaster of emotions. I just had to accept that the situation was hard and try to love and lead my wife well through it.

Maybe you've recently started to notice how waiting affects you as a husband. Infertility is your issue, too, not just your wife's struggle. Here are a few suggestions to help you depend on God and love your wife well.

We're in This Together

Beyond fixing the situation, something else that was not fixable were my wife's feelings. She didn't want me to fix her. She just needed to be heard, validated, supported, and to feel like we were doing this *together*. Believe it or not, letting her see that I was also falling apart at times brought us closer and made her feel like she wasn't alone. Infertility is a husband's issue, too, not just a woman's thing, regardless of whether there are medical issues involved with one or the other.

Men, I can't encourage you enough to actively take steps to show your wife that your heart hurts and to communicate your struggles. She needs to see both your strength and your weakness. This might mean you need to retrain your brain to not see vulnerability as weakness. It's perfectly okay to struggle together. Being completely without control over this situation forced me to rely on God's strength to sustain us.

There were moments when I wouldn't give Kelley the time she needed to talk about everything, because I thought that by changing the subject and talking about something else we could get her mind off it. But instead, this would make her feel isolated, like I didn't care enough to want to talk about it. I needed to provide her the space to communicate openly and honestly and do the same with her, to show her she wasn't alone in this journey.

Show Her You Care

Our wives can think that we don't care because we may not be as vocal about it or we may process things differently. Kelley and I experienced this in our own journey. Don't get me wrong—I cared the entire time and wanted to have kids, but at times I also cared about having back my happy wife whom I fell in love with and married.

There were times when my decisions and the words I said were probably more focused on trying to get back to normal, even if it meant putting off treatment for a little while. This made it seem like I didn't care about getting pregnant as much as she did and that I was okay with abandoning our pursuit of having children. It all came from a good place but caused conflict, because we have different points of view and I failed to communicate that effectively.

Ephesians 5:25 says, "Husbands, love your wives, just as Christ loved the church and gave himself up for her." I didn't have a problem loving her, but showing her that in tangible ways was at times a struggle for me. Weekly check-ins and being intentional with some of our time seemed to greatly help in showing that I cared about her and us. It was an open, safe place to share, engage, and help each other, and it kept us on the same page. During this journey there are a lot of times you simply aren't on the same page, with all the emotions, decisions, turns, and grieving going on in both of you. You must carve out time to work through the challenging situations together, to ensure you are unified. If you are the one who initiates this, she will be grateful to be supported and cared for.

Let Others In

I didn't know any other men going through this at the beginning of our infertility journey. But just because I didn't know other men specifically dealing with this did not mean I should avoid reaching out to other men I was close to for support. Men, fight the temptation to isolate, and let other people in.

It's likely your guy friends have heard that you and your spouse are in this difficult season, especially if your wife talks to other wives. Some of my guy friends mentioned that although they cared about us and wanted to support us, they were afraid to talk to me about it because they either thought I wouldn't want to talk about it or they were scared of saying something dumb.

Even though your close guy friends may not fully understand what you're going through, still reach out to them for prayer. It's important to open the door to the awkward conversation they're afraid to have with you for fear of not knowing what to say or how to support you.

Fight for Your Marriage

For us men, we've got to keep pursuing our wives as though we were still dating. Maybe even some dates when we don't talk about infertility at all. This is critical to reassure her that we love and desire her even when she is feeling inadequate and battling thoughts of not being able to provide a child for both of you to start your family. Even if you don't have children, you and your wife are still a family. Don't think you must have kids to be a family. This is important. Remember it and remind her of it.

Ultimately, if we forget about the importance of our relationship with our spouse during this tough season, we could end up with a child but also with a marriage that is falling apart. It is our responsibility as men to take the lead in making sure this doesn't happen. It can be easy for women to take the reins in the infertility journey, since so many decisions are happening in and about their bodies. But ultimately, we need to support, guide, and remind them that we are one and are in this together.

Although it takes a lot of work to make sure you have the relationship you had before infertility and come out even stronger, it is important. When Kelley and I were each selflessly focused on the other and worked at being friends on the same team, it was easier to choose to fight harder for what mattered: us.

Even in the most difficult times, we can trust that the parts of the Lord's will we don't want are the very things he'll use to accomplish his eternal plan. He is crafting, shaping, and planning at a much deeper level than we can see.

Helpful chapters for husbands include "Love Your Beloved," "Redeeming the Bedroom," "Should We Do IVF? (and Other Decisions)," "At What Cost?" and "Sighs of Sorrow" (if you've experienced a loss). Consider asking your wife if she would like to read any chapters together.

APPENDIX B

Help Me Wait

Dear family member, friend, or church leader,

Your relationship is important to me. I thank God for bringing you into my life and for the ways you've helped me grow. He created us for community, and I'm glad to belong to yours.

As you probably know, I'm walking through a hard season right now. Infertility, miscarriage, and waiting for a child affect every aspect of my life, including my relationship with you and other people. Because these are painful and complex experiences, it can be difficult for you to understand what I'm going through. You want to show me love, but you might feel confused, hesitant, or helpless. So I want to help you help me wait. Please listen to my suggestions, recognizing that everyone's journey is different. I promise to give you grace, and ask you to do the same for me.

Listen First

We often want to fill heavy silence with advice, a well-intentioned story, or even Scripture. But just be still. Wait. Listen. Let me fill the time and space when and how I'm able. I might want to vent about a difficult appointment, or simply have you hug me while I cry.

Be Sensitive

- Acknowledge my grief and the range of emotions I might be feeling.
- Resist the temptation to make assumptions. Don't assume that my husband and I haven't been trying to get pregnant "that long" or that our situation is just like someone else's you know or that we're not trusting God.
- Ask me how you can best offer support. I welcome questions such as, "Should I wait for you to update me?" or "May I call and ask you how your appointment went?" or "Would you want to be invited to the baby shower?"
- Set a reminder to pray for me and my husband on a regular basis.

Watch Your Words

- Don't give unsolicited advice. Unless I ask you to share, keep your personal experience and suggestions about what to try to yourself.
- Don't placate with false hope or Christian cliches. Examples include, "God will give you a baby"; "You'd be great parents"; "Just adopt"; "Go on vacation"; "I know it will happen for you"; "God will work it all out"; and "When God closes a door, he opens a window."
- Use open-ended questions and simple statements to communicate your concern: "How are you doing?" or "Would you mind if I pray for you now?" or "That's so hard."

Be Present

Your presence means more to me than anything you say. Small gestures like putting your hand on my shoulder when someone announces, "I'm pregnant!" give me comfort right when I need it. A member of our Waiting in Hope community shared, "My dear friend just texted that she would like to come over to sit with me. Just sit. I responded when I was ready and she honored that time. We sat on the porch, she squeezed my hand, and we both wept. It was exactly what I needed."

Love as a Church Family

The church is home for the family of believers. I'm sad to say I don't always feel like I belong in my home. Christians tend to elevate motherhood as a woman's greatest purpose. This brings an unintended consequence of making women like me feel overlooked, forgotten, and out of place.

As a church leader, you can point me to hope in Christ when you embrace me with the love of Christ. Take time to become educated about infertility, miscarriage, adoption, and other types of waiting for a child. Identify and acknowledge these struggles from the pulpit, especially on holidays, including Mother's Day and Father's Day. Consider hosting awareness events or special prayer gatherings specifically for couples facing infertility. Waiting in Hope can help you with this.

If someone in your congregation wants to start a Waiting in Hope support group, encourage her and offer to announce and/or publish the meeting in your bulletin. Think about devoting a time of prayer to lift up couples who are struggling to conceive and/or have lost babies through miscarriage. Your prayers make a difference and help me know that I'm seen and loved by my church family and thereby the Lord.

I Need You

Despite how complicated our relationship might be, I need you to bear this burden with me. God gave us one another to lean on for support. Thank you for sharing his comfort through your care.

APPENDIX C

About Waiting in Hope Ministries

Waiting in Hope Ministries is a biblical nonprofit support ministry founded by Kelley and Justin Ramsey in 2015, but it started in 2010 during their years of walking through infertility. The ministry aims to embrace, encourage, and support women and men facing infertility, miscarriage, adoption, and other types of waiting for a child.

Waiting in Hope Ministries recognizes God's call to minister through the local body of Christ. Our church partnership program equips local churches with curriculum, tools, and training to help them shepherd women and men who are suffering infertility in their congregations and communities. With more than a decade of infertility support experience, the Waiting in Hope team strives to collaborate with church partners to reach hurting hearts who need the light of the gospel. Each local support group gives women a compassionate space where they can grieve with others who understand the unique heartache of infertility. We train churches and leaders, helping them walk through the process of launching and maintaining a hope-filled community.

In addition to ongoing groups, Waiting in Hope Ministries hosts an annual couples retreat called *Waiting Well Together*. The retreat is a getaway designed to help couples rest, reconnect, and refocus their marriage on Christ during this challenging season of life.

Our online offerings include *Waiting in Hope Connection*, a private membership site. *Waiting in Hope Connection* provides a safe community where women and couples can find encouragement and resources without being exposed to the painful aspects of social media. Members can gain access to training courses, discussion forums, online events, and other resources.

We want to help women and men know they don't have to wait alone. Our greatest desire is to help them seek true and lasting hope in Jesus.

APPENDIX D

How to Put Your Faith in Jesus

Hope is why you're here. You picked up this book to find hope in your journey to have a baby. But your search for hope might have led you deeper than you expected. Maybe you sense there's something missing in your life—something more vital to your existence than a baby.

If your heart is stirring, we have amazing news for you. Jesus Christ died for you. He offered his own life to forgive you of every wrong you've ever done and will ever do. Though sin separated you from God, Jesus made you right with him, holy and perfect in his eyes.

God invites you to accept his gift of salvation through faith in his Son. These Bible verses can help you understand why we need Jesus:

1. All of us have sinned. (Romans 3:23)
2. The penalty for sin is death. (Romans 6:23)
3. God sent Jesus to take our place. (John 3:16)
4. If we confess our sins, he'll forgive us and wash away all our wrongs. (1 John 1:9)
5. Everyone who calls on the name of the Lord will be saved. (Romans 10:13)

This is the *gospel*, which means "good news." Jesus came to earth in human flesh, lived a perfect life, died on a cross, rose from the dead, and is enthroned as Lord over everything. When you believe in him, repent of your sins, and make him Lord of your life, he gives you peace with God and puts his Spirit within you.

If you've never prayed before, don't worry. God isn't looking for fancy words; he wants your heart. Here's a sample prayer to guide you:

Dear God, I'm a sinner and need forgiveness. I believe Jesus Christ shed his precious blood and died for my sins. I'm willing to turn from sin. I now put my faith in Christ and trust him as my Lord and Savior.

Welcome to your new, grace-transformed life! Be sure to tell a pastor or trusted family member or friend that you've accepted Jesus. We'd love to rejoice with you now that you have found Living Hope, so let us know by emailing hello@waitinginhopeinfertility.com.

Glossary

See the Waiting in Hope Ministries website (www.waitinginhopeinfertility.com /terminology) for more information on these words and phrases.[1]

Abnormal sperm: sperm with defects that may affect their ability to reach and penetrate an egg.

Clomid: medication used as a first-line fertility treatment to induce ovulation.

Ectopic pregnancy: when a fertilized egg implants and grows outside of the uterus, usually in a fallopian tube.

Embryo adoption: when a family adopts embryos remaining from a donor's in vitro fertilization, and the embryos are transferred to the adoptive mother's womb.[2]

Endometriosis: a condition where endometrial tissue grows outside the uterus, which can cause pain and infertility.

Human chorionic gonadotropin (HCG): hormone made by the placenta during pregnancy. Health-care providers look at HCG to confirm pregnancy and evaluate how a pregnancy is progressing.[3]

Hysteroscopy: procedure where a health-care provider checks the uterine lining and takes tissue samples as needed.[4]

Infertility: inability to conceive after a year of frequent, unprotected sex.

Intrauterine insemination (IUI): procedure in which sperm are placed in a woman's uterus at the time ovulation is expected.

In vitro fertilization (IVF): fertility treatment in which eggs and sperm are combined outside a woman's body in a laboratory. If fertilization happens, embryos are either transferred to her uterus or frozen for transfer later. Mini IVF involves the same process, but uses lower doses of egg stimulation medication.

Male factor infertility: caused by low sperm count, abnormal sperm shape or function, or physical problems that block sperm delivery.

Miscarriage: spontaneous loss of a pregnancy before the twentieth week of gestation.

Ovarian cysts: fluid-filled sacs in or on an ovary. Most ovarian cysts are harmless, but some can cause pain and affect the timing of a planned fertility treatment.

Ovulation: process in which a mature egg is released from the ovary. In normal conditions, the released egg moves down the fallopian tube where it can be fertilized by sperm.

Polycystic ovary syndrome (PCOS): hormonal imbalance that can lead to infrequent or longer menstrual cycles, which may cause infertility.

Premenstrual syndrome (PMS): symptoms that happen prior to menstruation, including mood swings, tender breasts, food cravings, fatigue, irritability, and depression.

Secondary infertility: when a woman can't get pregnant or carry a baby to term after having been pregnant before.

Stillbirth: death of a baby in the womb after twenty weeks' gestation or during delivery.[5]

Two-week wait (2WW): phrase describing how long a woman should wait to take a pregnancy test after sex, IUI, or IVF.

Unexplained infertility: when a couple can't get pregnant and no specific cause is found.

Notes

Chapter 3

1. Simone Biles (@Simone_Biles), Twitter, July 28, 2021, 8:46 p.m., https://twitter .com/Simone_Biles/status/1420561448883802118.
2. Brennan Manning, *Abba's Child* (Colorado Springs: NavPress, 1994), 51.

Chapter 4

1. Janet Jaffe, "Reproductive Trauma: Psychotherapy for Pregnancy Loss and Infertility Clients from a Reproductive Story Perspective," *Psychotherapy* 54, no. 4 (2017): 380–85, https://doi.org/10.1037/pst0000125.

Chapter 5

1. Ed Welch, *Shame Interrupted* (Greensboro: New Growth Press, 2012), 52.
2. Ibid.

Chapter 6

1. Uche Anadu Ndefo et al., "Polycystic Ovary Syndrome: a Review of Treatment Options with a Focus on Pharmacological Approaches," *P&T: A Peer-Reviewed Journal for Managed Care and Hospital Formulary Management* 38, no. 6 (2013): 336–55, https://www.ncbi.nlm.nih.gov/pmc/articles/PMC3737989/.
2. "Facts about endometriosis," Endometriosis.org, accessed July 6, 2022, https://endometriosis.org/resources/articles/facts-about-endometriosis/.

Chapter 8

1. To participate in our Waiting in Hope online community, visit waitinginhope infertility.com or join Waiting in Hope Chats at Facebook.com/groups /waitinginhopechats.

Chapter 9

1. Sarah R. Holley et al., "Prevalence and Predictors of Major Depressive Disorder for Fertility Treatment Patients and their Partners," *Fertility and Sterility* 103, no. 5 (May 2015): 1332–39, https://www.ncbi.nlm.nih.gov/pmc/articles/PMC4417384/.
2. Ellen W. Freeman et al., "Psychological Evaluation and Support in a Program of In Vitro Fertilization and Embryo Transfer," *Fertility and Sterility* 43, no. 1 (January 1985): 48–53, https://www.sciencedirect.com/science/article/pii/S0015028216483160.
3. Timothy Keller, *Walking with God through Pain and Suffering* (New York: Penguin Books, 2013), 121.

Chapter 10

1. Mark Vroegop, *Dark Clouds, Deep Mercy* (Wheaton: Crossway, 2019), 44.
2. Elisabeth Elliot, *Suffering Is Never for Nothing* (Nashville: B&H Publishing Group, 2019), 54.

Chapter 12

1. John Piper, "Worship: We Get Joy, God Gets Praise," Desiring God, June 26, 2017, https://www.desiringgod.org/messages/gospel-worship/excerpts/worship-we-get-joy-god-gets-praise.
2. A. W. Tozer, *The Knowledge of the Holy* (New York: HarperCollins, 1961), 1.

Chapter 14

1. John and Stasi Eldredge, *Captivating* (Nashville: Thomas Nelson, 2005), 84.

Chapter 17

1. "Infertility," Mayo Clinic, accessed July 6, 2022, https://www.mayoclinic.org/diseases-conditions/infertility/symptoms-causes/syc-20354317.
2. Joni Eareckson Tada, *A Lifetime of Wisdom* (Grand Rapids: Zondervan, 2009), 136.

Chapter 19

1. *Hebrew–English Dictionary,* s.v., "consider," https://hebrew.english-dictionary.help/english-to-hebrew-meaning-consider.

Chapter 20

1. Paul David Tripp, *Lost in the Middle* (Wapwallopen, Penn.: Shepherd Press, 2004), Kindle.

Chapter 21

1. Gary Thomas, *Sacred Marriage* (Grand Rapids: Zondervan, 2015), 1.

Chapter 22

1. Lise Brix, "Childless Couples Have More Divorces," February 11, 2014, ScienceNordic, https://sciencenordic.com/childbirth-denmark-divorce/childless -couples-have-more-divorces/1396768.

Chapter 23

1. To join our Waiting in Hope Chats, go to https://www.facebook.com/groups /waitinginhopechats/.

Chapter 25

1. Ann Voskamp, *The Broken Way* (Grand Rapids: Zondervan, 2016), 221.

Chapter 26

1. Charles Haddon Spurgeon, "Spiritual Knowledge and Its Practical Results," September 30, 1883, https://www.spurgeon.org/resource-library/sermons /spiritual-knowledge-and-its-practical-results/#flipbook/.

Chapter 27

1. Richard Rohr, *A Spring Within Us: A Year of Daily Meditations* (Sheridan: CAC Publishing, 2016), 199, 120–21.
2. "IVF Cost: Analyzing the True Cost of In Vitro Fertilization," CNY Fertility, November 26, 2021, https://www.cnyfertility.com/ivf-cost/.
3. "IVF—In Vitro Fertilization," Fertility IQ, accessed July 6, 2022, https://www .fertilityiq.com/ivf-in-vitro-fertilization/costs-of-ivf#cost-components.
4. "Cost of Adoption in the US," Creating a Family, accessed July 6, 2022, https://creatingafamily.org/adoption/resources/cost-adoption-us/.
5. Ibid.

6. "Program Fees and Financial Helps," Snowflakes, accessed July 6, 2022, https://nightlight.org/snowflakes-embryo-adoption-donation/embryo -adoption/funding/.

7. For more about Dave Ramsey's Financial Peace University, see https://www .ramseysolutions.com/store/digital-products/financial-peace-university-class.

Chapter 30

1. *Up*, screenplay by Bob Peterson and Pete Docter, Walt Disney Pictures, 2009.

2. For a biblical view on grieving childlessness, we recommend reading Chelsea Patterson Sobolik, *Longing for Motherhood: Holding on to Hope in the Midst of Childlessness* (Chicago: Moody Publishers, 2018).

3. *Up*, 2009.

4. Jill Briscoe, "The Mission Field is Between Your Feet," *100 Huntley Street*, accessed July 6, 2022, http://100huntley.com/watch?id=221906&title =the-mission-field-is-between-your-feet---jill-briscoe.

Chapter 31

1. Elisabeth Elliot, *Suffering Is Never for Nothing* (Nashville: B&H Publishing Group, 2019), 15.

Glossary

1. Unless otherwise noted, all glossary information found via "Diseases and Conditions," Mayo Clinic, accessed July 20, 2022, https://www.mayoclinic.org /diseases-conditions/.

2. "What Is Embryo Adoption?" Nightlight Christian Adoptions, accessed July 20, 2022, https://nightlight.org/snowflakes-embryo-adoption-donation/what -is-embryo-adoption/.

3. "Human Chorionic Gonadotropin," Cleveland Clinic, accessed July 20, 2022, https://my.clevelandclinic.org/health/articles/22489-human-chorionic -gonadotropin.

4. "Dilation and curettage (D&C)," Mayo Clinic, accessed July 20, 2022, https://www .mayoclinic.org/tests-procedures/dilation-and-curettage/about/pac-20384910.

5. "Stillbirth," Cleveland Clinic, accessed July 20, 2022, https://my.clevelandclinic .org/health/diseases/9685-stillbirth.

WAITING *in* HOPE

INFERTILITY SUPPORT MINISTRIES

WIH CONNECTION
ONLINE MEMBERSHIP COMMUNITY
created just for you with courses, events, and others to walk with

CHURCH PARTNERSHIPS
LOCAL SUPPORT GROUPS
start a group with proven curriculum, help, and training

WAITING WELL TOGETHER
COUPLES RETREAT
a purposeful getaway to refocus and strengthen marriages

WE CAN CHOOSE TO NOT SIMPLY WAIT
within our infertility,
BUT INSTEAD TO WAIT WITH HOPE!

FIND COMMUNITY | JOIN SUPPORT GROUP | FOLLOW US

Facebook.com/Waiting.in.Hope
waiting-in-hope-connection.mn.co
Instagram.com/waiting.in.hope

WAITINGINHOPEINFERTILITY.COM